UNDERSTANDING RADIOGRAPHY

By

STEPHEN S. HISS, R.T., C.X.T., B.S.

Administrative Technologist
Atlantic City Medical Center
Atlantic City, New Jersey

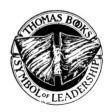

CHARLES C THOMAS · PUBLISHER
Springfield · Illinois · U.S.A.

Published and Distributed Throughout the World by
CHARLES C THOMAS • PUBLISHER
Bannerstone House
301-327 East Lawrence Avenue, Springfield, Illinois, U.S.A.

© *1978, by* CHARLES C THOMAS • PUBLISHER
ISBN 0-398-03685-3
Library of Congress Catalog Card Number: 77-8386

Library of Congress Cataloging in Publication Data
Hiss, Stephen S.
    Understanding radiography.

    Bibliography: p
    Includes index.
    1. Radiography, Medical—Image quality
    2. Radiography, Medical—Processing.   I. Title.
[DNLM: 1. Technology, Radiologic.   2. Radiography.
WN160 H673u]
RC78.H52   616.07'572   77-8386
ISBN 0-398-03685-3

Printed in the United States of America
P-4

To my wife Patricia
who sacrificed much during the preparation of this volume
and to my daughter Kimberly
for her innocent love

FOREWORD

After a long wait, an up-to-date, complete, and well researched text on radiography has been written, published, and is available to student radiological technologists. Experienced technologists should also be made aware of this text because of the new approaches presented and the current information it contains.

The format is excellent and takes one, in a well organized and easily understandable manner, from the basic concepts regarding the characteristics of the radiographic image through to the more advanced ideas involving practical x-ray physics without the pitfalls of cumbersome and difficult language. The chapter on conversions is excellent and should provide the reader with a very workable foundation from which adjustments can be made regarding exposure factors. The final chapter very skillfully leads the reader into a discussion of film critique and gives a very practical approach to critiquing a radiograph that is certain to prove beneficial in everyday radiography for all practicing technologists.

The author has done an outstanding job in bringing to light important factors that are sure to offer not only food for thought, but in addition, a well organized and thorough discussion of the important concepts that have not, until now, been fully developed.

The illustrations are also well done, interesting, and very informative. The radiographs used are of excellent quality and, for the first time, the reader and instructor can actually see and appreciate the message they carry.

From an instructor's point of view, the style with which the text is written is easy to understand and will easily hold the reader's attention.

I believe this text will prove to be an outstanding contribution to the field of radiological technology.

RAYMOND HORNER, R.T., F.A.S.R.T.
Harrisburg Poly Clinic
Harrisburg, Pennsylvania

PREFACE

D URING the early planning stages of this text, a few important prerequisites were self-imposed in the firm belief that their absence would yield a publication so similar to those presently available that another text simply would not be justified. The information presented within the following pages is in some instances new ground for even the experienced technologist while, in other instances, old familiar concepts have been reassessed and aligned more closely with current data.

An important goal which had been set is that strict attention and ample time would be given to the many aspects of radiography which have, in the past, been treated perhaps too simplistically. Although complex physical formulae are not contained in this volume, an attempt has been made to not merely present these concepts of modern radiography for purposes of identification, but also to discuss and analyze each issue at hand from more than one perspective. Without this more rounded approach, much of the meaning is often lost, and as a result misconceptions and frustrations take the place of enlightenment.

It has been my intention from the outset that the information within these pages be presented in such a way that it can be readily understood, and that each concept discussed is covered thoroughly enough and with sufficient depth that an accurate insight can be gained to bridge the gap students often feel is present between classroom theory and its practical application.

In the end, it is often the concept of an idea that is most important to remember, because from it one can learn to answer many of his own questions.

The primary intention of this text is to provide those concepts and insights from which the technologist can grow into a competent professional.

S.S.H.

ACKNOWLEDGMENTS

No undertaking of this type can be accomplished without a considerable amount of encouragement, conversation, advice, and reliable facts. Those individuals who have freely given their knowledge regarding radiography have my warmest and deepest appreciation: A great deal of thanks is heartily given to Mr. Thomas Callear, Mr. Edward Cook, Mr. Lee Erickson, and Mr. Robert Trinkle for their hours of time, valued information, and advice.

A number of commercial representatives also freely gave time from their busy schedules to help me obtain data I would not have otherwise been able to present in these pages. In appreciation for their individual efforts, I would like to thank Mr. Donald Becker, Mr. James Funk, Mr. Gary Goodridge, Mr. Harry Harter, Mr. William Orledge, Mr. Gene Oxley, Mr. Tony Passarelli, Mr. Lin Tiley, and Mr. James Wagner.

I would like to also express my thanks to Mr. B. Gilman Cutting for his help and suggestions.

Much appreciation is given to those who helped in proofreading the typed manuscript. Their opinions and comments weighed heavily in the final preparation of this text. For their effort, I would like to thank Ms. Rosann Allen, Ms. Cathy Blose, Ms. Veronica Brodovicz, Ms. Lynda Callaway, Mr. Ernest Griffith, Ms. Catherine Harbaugh, Ms. Mary Matas, Ms. Joann Newell, and Ms. Deborah Wolf.

I would also like to thank Mr. Michael Martinchick for his time in preparing the negatives used in the text, and for his skill, sincere encouragement, and concern for the success of this writing.

I wish to thank Dr. Albert Salzman, Dr. Sigmond Rutkowski, and the Associates in Radiology for making available important radiographs from the teaching library of the Division of Radiology at The Atlantic City Medical Center. I would also like to thank Mr. Charles Broomall, Administrator at A.C.M.C., for his help and consideration.

Sincere thanks must be given to Mr. Jonathan Law for his interest and effort, and for the information he gave freely.

There are moments in one's career when a single choice must be made regarding the direction of one's career. Mr. Frank Horvath will never be forgotten for the opportunity he afforded by introducing me to radiography and for his unselfish guidance, good will, and trust.

Mr. Jack Cullinan's help and treasured advice have given me a wealth of knowledge and insight into radiography. His thoughtfulness, knowledge, and good will cannot be properly expressed in words, only felt within.

For the help and long hours spent printing the negatives to meet high standards, I very much want to thank Mr. Leroy Knupp, Ocean City Camera Shop, Ocean City, New Jersey.

The illustrations in this text were provided by Ms. Sue Criss. Her talent and cooperation in their preparation are indeed appreciated.

For the opportunity to work with a publisher who expresses sincere interest in the author's well-being without sacrificing quality, I wish to thank Mr. Payne Thomas. His attitude throughout this project was one of support, trust, and the provider of valued guidance. To Mr. Thomas and his staff at Charles C Thomas, Publisher, I wish to express my sincere appreciation for their help and effort.

Mrs. Patricia Donnon deserves a great deal of thanks for laboring through my first set of handwritten notes and putting them into the first typing. Untold hours must have been spent deciphering those scribblings.

In the long run, good will and trust often determine the success of an undertaking. For those gifts I wish to thank my parents, Nicholas and Sophia.

S.S.H.

CONTENTS

Chapter   *Page*

One   **Characteristics Of The Radiographic Image** 3

Radiographic Balance 3

Radiographic Contrast 6

Elements of Radiographic Contrast....................... 8

Why Different Film Contrasts Are Used.................. 10

Radiographic Density 12

Elements of Radiographic Density....................... 12

Visibility versus Sharpness of Detail....................... 15

Sharpness of Detail 16

Visibility of Detail 16

Sensitometry 18

The Location of The H & D Curve....................... 21

The Shape of The H & D Curve......................... 21

Film Latitude 22

Film Contrast 24

Determining Film Contrast from The H & D Curve......... 25

Base Plus Fog 26

Two   **Radiographic Film** 27

Film Manufacturing, an Art............................... 27

Various Types of Film Composition....................... 27

The Film Base 30

Film Base Characteristics 30

Base Thickness and Parallex Distortion................. 31

Base Plus Fog 32

Silver Bromide Crystals 32

Crystal Size, Quantity, and Shape...................... 32

Crystal Size and Radiographic Contrast................. 34

Film Contrast and Latitude............................ 35

The Gelatin 35

The Effect of Double Film Coating...................... 36

Film Storage 37

Latent Image Formation 37

Chapter		Page
	The Crystal Lattice	38
	Developer and Fixer Solutions	43
	Processing Solutions	44
	Chemical Fog	46
Three	**Automatic Processing**	47
	Introduction	47
	Centralized Versus Dispersal Processing	48
	Early Automatic Processors	49
	Some Important Considerations for Automatic Processing	51
	Major Systems in Automatic Processors	53
	The Transport System	53
	The Margin of Error	54
	The Crossover Assembly	55
	Artifacts Commonly Linked to The Transport System	56
	The Replenishment System	57
	Overreplenishment	57
	Underreplenishment	62
	Setting Replenishment Rates	64
	The Drying System	65
	Drying Problems	66
	The Recirculating System	66
	Troubleshooting Processor Problems	69
	Explanation	69
	Dark Films	71
	Light Films, Poor Contrast	71
	Films Have a Brownish Look	72
	Films Have a Milky Look	72
	Films Have a Greasy Look	72
	Jamming	72
	Scratches	73
	Black, Flaky Marks	73
	Increased Fog	73
	Routine Maintenance	74
	Sensitometric Strips	74
Four	**Intensifying Screens**	76
	General Construction	77
	Backing	77

Chapter		Page
	The Reflective Layer	78
	The Active Layer	80
	The Edge Seal	80
	The Process of Light Emission	80
	Fluorescence	81
	Phosphorescence	83
	Other Important Crystal Characteristics	83
	Classification of Screens	84
	The Practicality of Having Different I.F.s	86
	How Do Screens Affect The Radiographic Image?	86
	Contrast and Density	86
	Screen Sharpness	87
	Modulation Transfer Function	87
	Factors Affecting Screen Speed	93
	Screen Artifacts	97
	Quantum Mottle (Noise)	103
	Rare Earth Screens	103
	Maintenance of Screens	105
	Nonscreen Versus Screen Film	109
Five	**Milliamperage**	110
	Definition and Function	110
	The X-ray Tube Filament	111
	Ma, Heat, Focal Spot Size, and Radiographic Sharpness	115
	Reciprocity Law	115
	Milliamperage Calibration	117
	Patient Dose and Milliamperage	119
	The Radiographic Effect	122
	Density and Milliamperage	122
	Contrast and Milliamperage	123
	Exposure Time	125
	Exposure Time and The X-ray Beam	127
	Exposure Time and Scatter Radiation	128
	Automatic Timing Devices	128
Six	**Focal Film Distance**	133
	Introduction	133
	The Geometric Beam (or Fragment Beam)	133
	Focal Film Distance and The Inverse Square Law	134

Chapter *Page*

Focal Film Distance and Radiographic Contrast 137
   Choosing The Correct F.F.D. 137
The Line Focus Principle 141
   The Point Source 142
   Focal Spot Size 144
   Three Ways to Control Penumbra 144
Object Film Distance and Magnification 152
   The Magnification Technique 157
   Prerequisite for Magnification Technique 158
   Object Film Distance and Scatter Radiation 163
   Additional Advantages in Using Increased Object Film
      Distance 164
Distortion of The Radiographic Image 165
   Shape Distortion 165
   Size Distortion 165
   Stereotaxis Procedures 168
   The Heel Effect 170

Seven   **Kilovoltage** 174
Definition and Function 174
   Kilovoltage, Tube Current, and The X-ray Tube 175
   Kilovoltage and The X-ray Circuit 177
Beam Quantity and Quality 178
   Kilovoltage and Beam Quality 179
   Wave Length Distribution 179
   Kilovoltage and Subject Contrast 182
Exposure Latitude and Kilovoltage 184
   Kilovoltage, Patient Dose, and Beam Efficiency 188
Kilovoltage and Scatter Production 191
   Kilovoltage, Radiographic Density, and Contrast 193
   Fixed Versus Variable KvP Techniques 197

Eight   **The Human Body As An Emitter And Beam Modifier** 200
Major Absorbers of The Body 201
   Some General Facts Regarding Body Habitus 202
   Fat Content 204
   Muscle Content 207
   Water Content 212
   Bone Content 212

Chapter		*Page*

Evaluating The Patient 214
Important Characteristics of Major Body Regions 217
The Chest Region 217
The Abdomen 217
The Extremities 219
The Skull 220
A Look at Photon-Tissue Interactions 221
Photoelectric Interaction 221
Compton Interaction 227
Summary 229
Filtration and Radiography 229
The Radiographic Effect of Filtration 230

Nine **Controlling The Remnant Beam** 235
The Concept of Coning 235
Types of Beam-Limiting Devices 235
Basic Construction of a Collimator 236
Uses for Conventional Coning 240
The Radiographic Effect of Beam-Limiting Devices 240
Influences on Patient Dose 242
Summary 242
Radiographic Grids 243
The Concept 243
Construction 244
Grid Ratio 244
Grid Cutoff 247
Stereo Radiography 248
High Ratio Grids and Cutoff 249
Major Types of Grids 249
Nonfocused and Focused Grids 249
Cross Hatch Grids 253
Linear Versus Cross Grids 256
Lead Content 260
Moving Grids 260
Types of Bucky Assemblies 260
Grids and The General Radiographic Effect 261
Radiographic Density 261
Selecting The Proper Grid 263
Scatter Radiation 263

Chapter   *Page*

     Kilovoltage 263
     Body Part 265
    The Environment 266
     Focal Film Distance 267
     Grid Cassettes 267
   Summary 269

Ten   **Tomography** 270
   Why Do We Use Tomography? 270
    The Basic Concept 270
   Making Adjustments for Cut Thickness 275
   Excursion Speed 276
   Types of Excursion Patterns 281
   The Book Cassette and Multiplanography 283
   Thick Versus Thin Cuts 287
   Zonography 287
   Choosing a Starting Point 289
    Establishing Exposures for Tomography 293
    Types of Linkages 293
    Pluridirectional Tomography 298
    Balancing Exposure Factors for Tomography 299
    The Selection of Amplitude 299

Eleven **Conversion Factors In Radiography** 303
   Conversion Factors 313

Twelve **Film Critique** 323
   Visibility and Definition of Detail 326
    The Effect of Contrast on Visibility of Detail 326
    Sharpness of Detail 329
   An Approach to Film Critique 330
    How to Identify a Definition Problem 332
     Causes for Blurring 333
    Causes of Problems in Visibility of Detail 333
    The Correct Procedure 338
    An Approach to Film Critique 338
    Trouble Shooting the Radiographic Image 340

Bibliography 349

Index 351

UNDERSTANDING RADIOGRAPHY

CHAPTER ONE

CHARACTERISTICS OF THE RADIOGRAPHIC IMAGE

THE TERM RADIOGRAPH is most commonly used to identify a permanent image produced by x-rays; however, over the years, terms such as *roentgenogram* or *plate* have been used to identify the permanent image. *Roentgen,* of course, is taken from Wilhelm Roentgen's discovery of x rays, and *plates* was used because the first permanent images were on pieces of plate glass that had been coated with a silver bromide emulsion.

RADIOGRAPHIC BALANCE

The radiographic image must meet certain requirements to be of any medical value, and although the standards are considerably higher today than they were at some point earlier in time, the specific characteristics desired have not changed. Considering all the desirable properties an image should possess (see Fig. 1), technical balance is perhaps the most important. In a radiographic sense, balance is the relationship between contrast, density, and sharpness. It would be incorrect, however, to associate a specific contrast with a specific density, or sharpness. A balanced radiograph can have short or long scale contrast and can be light or dark. This is an important concept for the technologist to realize because if he can learn to identify a technically imbalanced image he will more easily know when to make technical adjustments or corrections. Figure 2 shows

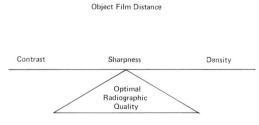

Figure 1. Contrast and density must compliment each other in order to produce optimal radiographic results. Too much or too little contrast for a given density or vice versa will destroy radiographic quality.

[3]

the diagnostic value of a well-balanced radiographic image as compared to one that is not. An imbalanced image may also be too flat or too light, and detail that one ordinarily expects to be present will be absent. It is

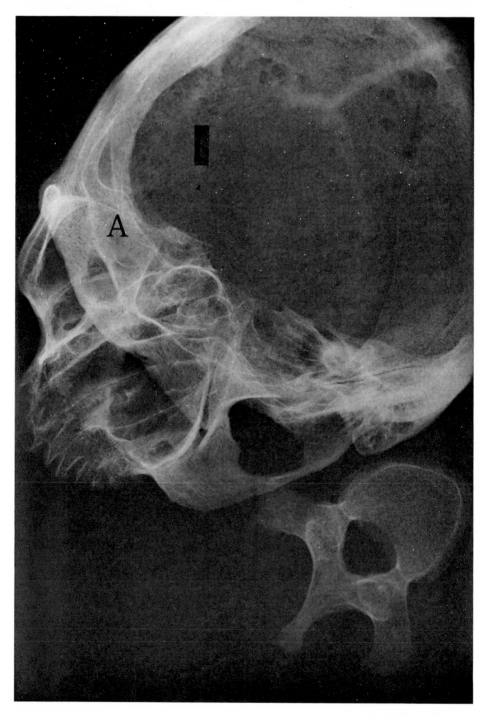

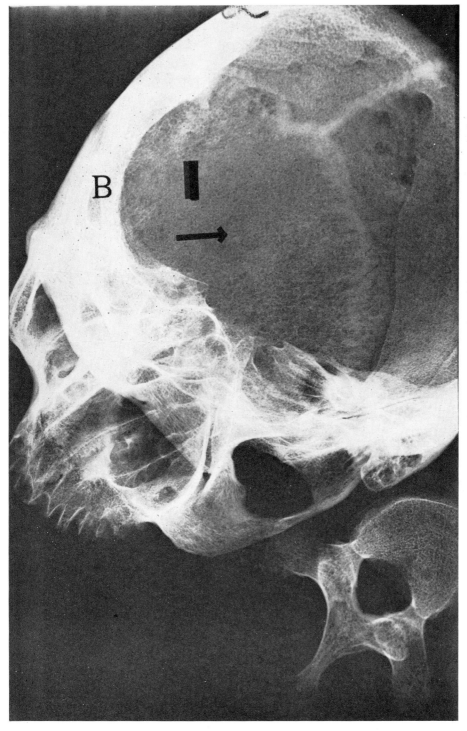

← Figure 2. Visibility of detail is much improved from *A* to *B* as a result of improved density.

important that such characteristics as these be identified as separate entities by the technologist so that he will have a basis from which corrections can be made. The author's feeling is that a technologist who cannot appreciate the quality or lack of it in a radiographic image will not be able to affect the appropriate adjustments necessary to correct the problem.

In summary, one can state that overall technical quality of a radiographic image is strongly dependent upon the compatibility that exists between contrast, density, and sharpness, and, if one is not dominant over the other, a certain technical balance has been successfully achieved. Later in the text, much discussion and evidence will be presented as to how such a balance can be obtained by using the various tools the technologist has at his disposal.

Radiographic Contrast

The amount of effort it takes to produce a radiographic image is of no importance if suitable radiographic contrast cannot be achieved; it is the

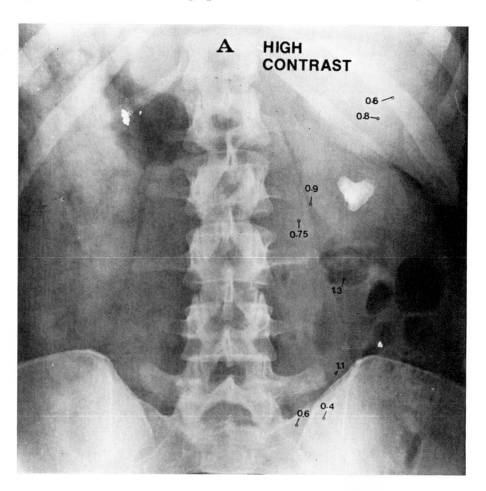

variations in density (contrast) that produce visibility of detail. Even in a nonradiographic sense, we cannot see any distinguishing parts if some type of contrast is missing. For example, upon looking at a solid green wall we will experience great difficulty in seeing any kind of detailed structures that are also green in color. However, if the various structures, cracks, curves, or chip marks are painted blue their presence is noted immediately. Similarly, if a radiograph exhibits only one tone, it is impossible to distinguish any body structures in the image. Fortunately, the radiographic image is composed of millions of tiny black silver crystals that, when viewed with the naked eye, form a pattern of different densities. Figure 3 shows a radiograph of an abdomen in which we see many dif-

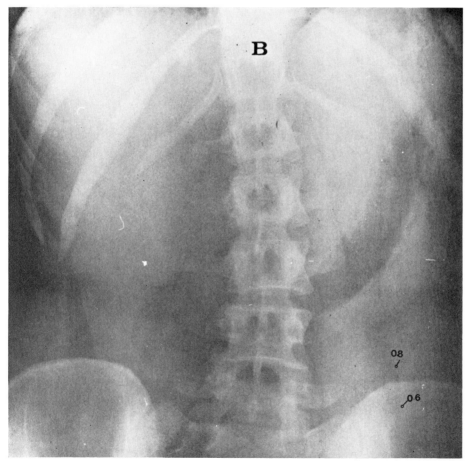

← Figure 3. In *A* the radiographic contrast is sufficient to easily demonstrate the various body parts. The overall density allows for optimal visualization as well. If the densities in *A* and *B* are compared in the pelvic region, the value of radiographic contrast can be understood. There is good sharpness as the borders of the various structures are well defined. *A* is indeed a well-balanced radiograph.

ferent shades of gray, each representing a body structure. Some of the shades (or tones) have been given actual numerical values. The kidneys, for example, can usually be seen, and it should be pointed out that the only reason we can distinguish their presence in the radiograph is that they display a slightly different density than do the structures in their immediate surroundings. As we scan the abdomen and look at the inferior areas of the liver where the gallbladder is located, no such distinction can be made because the gallbladder has the same density as the tissue around it. The pelvic bone is easily distinguished in the radiograph because the space it occupies in the film is a different density than its surroundings. In general, one can say that it is the difference in radiographic tones (densities) that produces contrast, and the ease with which a body part can be seen in the radiographic image is dependent on the *degree* of contrast present between its own tone or density and that of the body part or area around it. The various densities (see Fig. 3) in film B are closer in relationship than those in film A. The simple formula noted below is used to illustrate actual contrast values.

$$2^D - 1^D = \text{Contrast}$$

In Figure 4, the contrast values for A and B in the areas measured are noted; compare with C and D. The reason why the various densities can be produced in the image is that as x-ray photons pass through the body they are randomly absorbed by the various body parts. This differential absorption within the body causes the *exiting* photons to carry that absorption pattern on to the film as demonstrated in Figure 5. The x-ray film in this regard acts something like a mirror: it responds to the various intensities of the remnant photons emerging from the patient as a result of random tissue absorption. This aspect of radiography is known as subject contrast, which is extremely important and will be given proper attention later in the text. So far we have said in essence that radiographic contrast is the difference in density between two or more tones and that such contrast can be measured by subtracting density A from density B. Also, it was pointed out that unless sufficient contrast exists in an image, no diagnostic information of value can be seen. We will now go on to cover some of the important factors that contribute to overall radiographic contrast.

Elements of Radiographic Contrast

There are actually two major elements that make up radiographic contrast: subject contrast and film contrast. Subject contrast is the amount of differential absorption that has taken place among the various body structures lying in the path of the x-ray beam. The more pronounced these

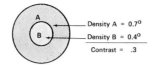

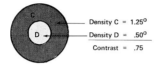

(As With The X-Ray Image These Densities Were Produced Only
With Changing The Number Of Black Specks Per M.M. Area)

Figure 4.

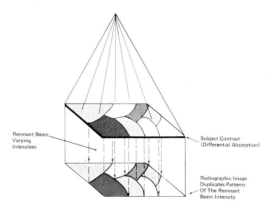

Figure 5. There is a direct relationship between subject contrast, film contrast, and radiographic contrast.

absorption differences are, the greater the subject contrast will be (see Fig. 6, which shows that the radiographic contrast is greatest between A and B). Other things remaining constant, the degree of differential absorption (subject contrast) will determine radiographic contrast. As subject contrast is increased, radiographic contrast will increase; as subject contrast decreases, radiographic contrast will decrease (assuming all the factors are held constant).

A certain harmony or compatibility must exist between subject contrast and film contrast. Film contrast denotes the inherent sensitivity a given emulsion has to variations in the intensity of remnant photons striking its surface. This sensitivity is manufactured into the film and can be increased and decreased by the manufacturer according to the requirements of the radiologist and technologist. Figure 7 shows two radio-

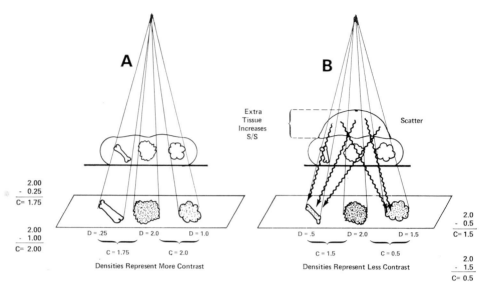

Figure 6. As x-rays are absorbed to different degrees, a corresponding pattern is produced by the film.

graphs of the same patient taken with the same exposure but using different film; by reviewing the radiographs carefully, you will note that film (A) has produced a greater degree of contrast than (B). The determining factor in this case is the film's own ability to emphasize the varying intensities of remnant photons striking the film. Thus, it can be correctly stated that if subject contrast (S.C.) and scatter (S/S) are held constant, film contrast controls radiographic contrast. This can be summarized as follows:

$\blacktriangle$ S.C. $\underset{x'}{\underset{x}{+}}$ (fixed film contrast) = $\blacktriangle$ radiographic contrast
$\blacktriangledown$ S.C. $+$ (fixed film contrast) = $\blacktriangledown$ radiographic contrast
(Fixed S.C.) $\underset{y}{+}$ $\blacktriangle$ film contrast = $\blacktriangle$ radiographic contrast
(Fixed S.C.) $\underset{x}{+}$ $\blacktriangledown$ film contrast = $\blacktriangledown$ radiographic contrast

Why Different Film Contrasts are Used

Students may ask why film is manufactured with different sensitivities to the remnant beam. The answer is that a harmony must exist between film and subject contrast before a good radiographic result can be gained. There is indeed an optimum radiographic contrast for different body parts which will best demonstrate *that* particular area, and it is the responsibility of film contrast to help produce this optimum condition for the viewer.

For example, the chest region has a great degree of subject contrast; if a high contrast film were used to record this area of the body, the re-

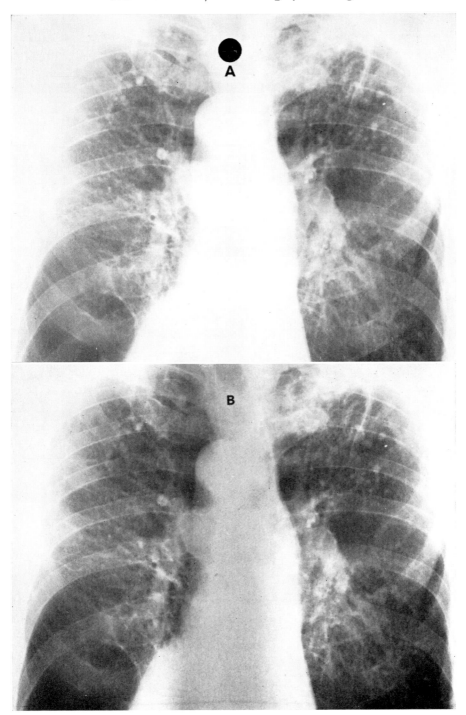

Figure 7. Given the same conditions, the film's inherent ability to emphasize intensities of the remnant beam will determine radiographic contrast. The film used for *B* was a low contrast film.

sulting radiographic contrast might be outside this optimum range (too much radiographic contrast). Likewise breast tissue has an extremely low subject contrast because the differential absorption of the structures is very low; if a low contrast film were used to record that particular body part, an extremely low radiographic contrast would result and would be below the optimal range for diagnosis. With this in mind, one can more readily understand the purpose of manufacturing various film contrasts: Various body regions cause different absorption abilities, and x-ray film is a sufficient variable to complement subject contrast or modify its effect to produce the desired radiographic contrast for good visualization of detail.

There are many factors that in turn contribute to film contrast and subject contrast. For example, it was stated that film contrast is the inherent ability of a film to record varying intensities of the x-ray photons exiting the patient, but it is generally held that processing is an important factor in film contrast. It will be discussed in Chapters Two and Three how different chemical activities and developing solution temperatures affect film contrast. When film contrast is mentioned, one should mentally include processing as well.

Subject contrast in itself is complex and involves such factors as body thickness, density, atomic number of the structure under examination, and kilovoltage.

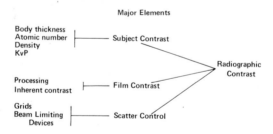

Radiographic Density

There must be an overall density present in the radiographic image to produce optimal detail visualization. Density is obtained when a sufficient *accumulation* of black metallic silver crystals is present in the film; this accumulation of silver is directly related to the number of remnant photons that struck the film during an exposure. If a small number of x-ray photons strike the film, the accumulation of black silver crystals will be sparse and when the film is placed on the x-ray illuminator, the eye will have great difficulty seeing the intended detail. However, if a remnant beam is sufficiently intense, the overall accumulation of silver would be evident along with associated detail. In Figure 8 two circles have been drawn with different image densities. Circle A produces an image of low density as compared to B. The only reason these circles appear different is that there are more dots per square inch in B (the dots themselves are the same size); they represent deposits of black silver.

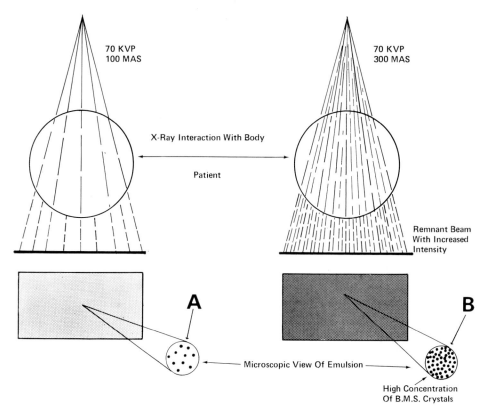

Figure 8. The degree of blackness (density) in a radiographic image is the specific result of how concentrated the black metallic crystals in the film's emulsion are after processing.

	A	B
Exposure =	2,000 photons	4,000 photons
Absorption =	1,000	2,000
Remnant photons =	1,000	2,000
Radiographic Density =	may be 1.0	may be 2.0

Elements of Radiographic Density

Radiographic density like radiographic contrast is the result of a combination of factors. The two major factors are film speed (which includes processing) and sufficient quantities of remnant photons. X-ray film man-

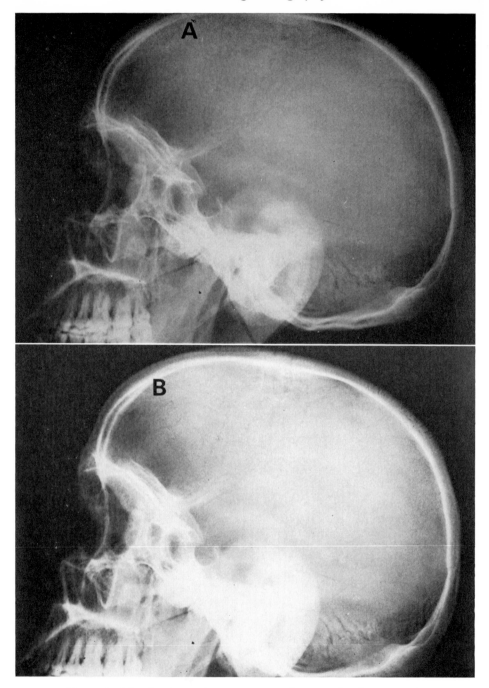

Figure 9. The density in *A* is approximately twice the density in *B*.

ufacturers have developed an ability to "give" x-ray film not only the sensitivity to record *varying intensities* (film contrast) but also an overall sensitivity to x-rays. The sensitivity a film has to x-ray photons or light from intensifying screens is known as film speed, and it has a strong influence on overall radiographic density. In the above example, the radiographic density in A was given as 1.0. However, if another type of x-ray film were used with the same exposure, a density perhaps of 2.0 may result because the inherent sensitivity of the second film to a given intensity of x-ray photons is greater and will respond more dramatically to the exposure. Stated more concisely, for a given intensity of remnant photons, the second film will produce more black silver because of its increased sensitivity. Figure 9 shows two different speed films taken under equal exposure and processing conditions. Film speed is primarily affected by the manufacturers ability to control emulsion thickness and crystal size.

In summary, radiographic density is the degree of blackness over the area being viewed and it is determined by the film's speed and the quantity of *remnant* radiation striking the film.

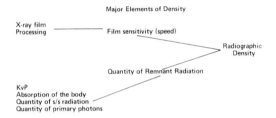

VISIBILITY VERSUS SHARPNESS OF DETAIL

In addition to radiographic contrast and density, the desired result is to see the various body structures with maximum sharpness. Sharpness or definition is the third major image characteristic. The radiographic image actually has two types of detail: (1) visibility of detail and (2) sharpness of detail. If the technologist can develop a clear distinction between these forms of detail, he will have a good start in reaching his goal of understanding radiography. Figure 10 is a schematic drawing of an x-ray tube emitting a primary beam. As the primary beam passes through the object under examination and proceeds to the film as remnant radiation, it produces a geometric pattern much the way a shadow of a tree is produced by the sun's rays. You will note that x-ray film records a "geometric impression" into its emulsion as shown, and also a pattern of contrast and densities. Thus, the radiographic image is actually a composite of two distinctly different entities, one being responsible for producing sharpness

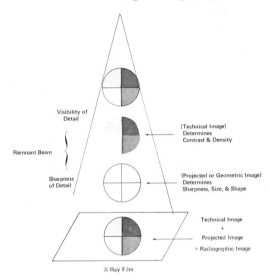

Figure 10. A remnant beam is actually composed of two distinct entities, the technical image (contrast and density) and the geometric image (sharpness). These components can be altered by the technologist independently of each other.

and the other being responsible for providing sufficient density and contrast. Those items that have an effect on sharpness or definition are said to control definition of detail and those items that effect radiographic contrast and density have control over visibility of detail.

Sharpness of Detail

The projected x-ray beam (or projected image) is primarily responsible for producing sharpness of detail, and anything that alters the projected beam will alter sharpness of the image. There are many things that influence definition of detail, and they will be covered in Chapter Six. In short, they are focal spot size, focal film distance, object film distance, screens, and motion.

Visibility of Detail

Visibility of detail is something quite different. As sharpness of detail is controlled by the geometry of the projected beam, visibility of detail is how well we can see the structures that have been transferred to the film's emulsion by the quantity and variation of remnant photons.

In Figure 11, the overall radiographic detail is poor because the image is too dark and because contrast is poor, so visibility of detail is poor. An analogy can be used to help explain this concept: If one looks at a tall building at a distance, it can be seen rather easily; the sharp borders of the building are also distinguished. However, if a fog bank would move into the area, the geometric dimensions of the building would not be

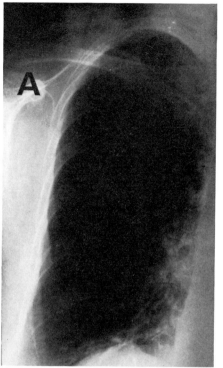

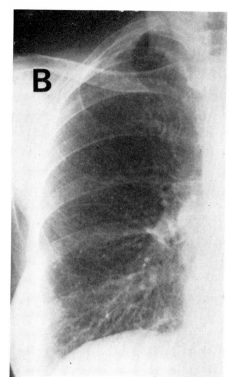

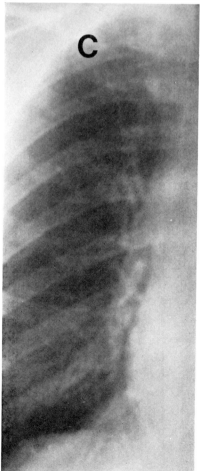

Figure 11. Visibility of detail (contrast and density) must be adequate to *see* various body structures. *A* has optimal sharpness which cannot be fully appreciated because of excessive density. *B* shows correct density. *C* shows poor sharpness but good density and contrast.

visible. This certainly is not because the structure is no longer present, but because something occurred that obstructed its *visibility.* If the same building is viewed on a clear night, the building once again is not visible, although the geometric structure of the building is present. In this instance, the building is not visible because of blackness of the night. It is important that the technologist can distinguish these two forms of detail. If one recognizes a radiograph that exhibits poor visibility of detail he need only work to correct those factors that can affect visibility of detail.

If radiographic detail is poor because of a geometric problem, only the factors that control the projection are to be corrected and not those related to visibility of detail.

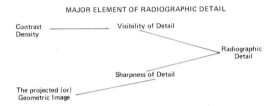

MAJOR ELEMENT OF RADIOGRAPHIC DETAIL

Contrast
Density
Visibility of Detail

Radiographic
Detail

Sharpness of Detail

The projected (or)
Geometric Image

SENSITOMETRY

Sensitometry is the process of giving quantitative values to the image characteristics of contrast, latitude, and density and also the arrangement of their values into a logical form or chart that can be easily analyzed. Figure 12 shows two gray scales with actual density values indicated. The numbers were obtained from readings made by an instrument known as a densitometer. The device is very sensitive to various levels of light and will give numerical readings to each density tone it is presented with. From the general appearance of the two scales, it is quite obvious they are different, yet unless we use the densitometer, it is difficult to put these scales into workable terms for comparison purposes.

A graph could be used to display these values, which would furnish much more information. In Figure 13, the vertical scale measures the degree of density a particular film was able to produce and the horizontal scale gives the amount of radiation that was required to produce that density. Figure 14 shows how the two gray scales would appear if translated into a chart known as an H & D curve. The dots indicating density levels are then connected to form a curve that when interpreted shows some important characteristics of the film being tested. Further, it should be noted that H & D curves are broken into three major sections with dividing points shown below.

$$\text{Toe} = 0^D \text{ to } 0.25^D$$
$$\text{Body} = 0.25^D \text{ to } 2.0^D$$
$$\text{Shoulder} = 2.1^D \text{ to maximum reading}$$

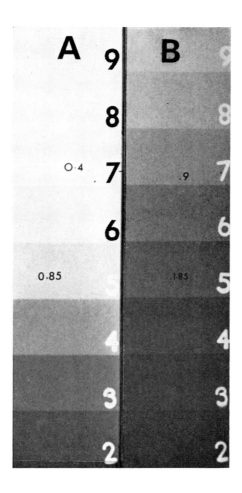

Figure 12. A gray scale of densities is depicted: *A* is a high or short scale, *B* is a low or long scale.

As you view the curves in Figure 14 it is evident that they have various shapes and also occupy different areas of the chart. These two factors in essence provide a technologist with all necessary information regarding the film's contrast, speed, and latitude characteristics.

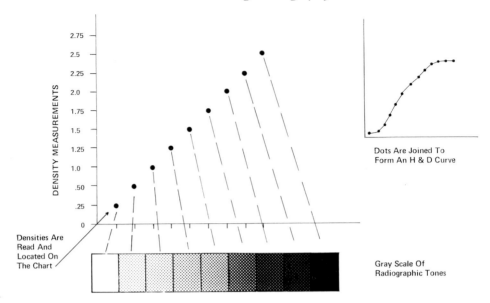

DENSITY MEASUREMENTS

Densities Are
Read And
Located On
The Chart

Dots Are Joined To
Form An H & D Curve

Gray Scale Of
Radiographic Tones

Figure 13.

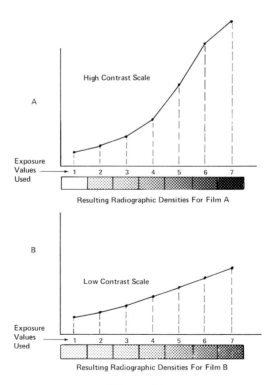

A

High Contrast Scale

Exposure
Values
Used

Resulting Radiographic Densities For Film A

B

Low Contrast Scale

Exposure
Values
Used

Resulting Radiographic Densities For Film B

Figure 14.

The Location of the H & D Curve

Location refers to how far toward the left or right the body of the curve appears on the chart. In Figure 15, we see two curves at various locations. Curves are tangent lines which can present a problem for interpretation because density readings vary along the curve from one point to another. With this in mind, 1^D was agreed upon to be used as a fixed reference point. For example, in the body in curve A, 1^D is located far to

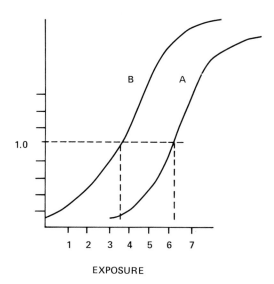

Figure 15. The left to right location or position of the curve, at D^1, is used to determine speed.

the right side of the chart. Keeping in mind that the numbers along the horizontal scale indicate quantity of exposure, we can see that much more exposure was needed before film (A) produced enough black metallic silver to reach a density of 1^D. On the other hand, in film (B), less exposure was needed to make a density of 1^D. Thus, by using the location or lateral position of a curve, the technologist knows that (A) is much less sensitive to x-rays and therefore is termed a slow film, certainly slower than film (B). If you examined the relative exposure values that were used to produce a density of 1, you would find that one-half the exposure was required to produce the same amount of film density in film (B), showing that (B) is twice as fast as film (A).

The Shape of the H & D Curve

Within reason, the position or location of the curve can fall anywhere on the chart, but it should be pointed out that location has no relevance to its shape (shape means the overall appearance or form of the curve).

Figure 16 shows three curves at approximately the same position on the chart; from a theoretical point of view, all three films have the same speed because 1ᴰ was obtained with the same exposure values, yet the curves are different in other ways. Film (1) has a very vertical body with a sudden fattening at the shoulder and toe. Film (2) produced a curve that has a more moderate angle and with a more subtle change at the shoulder and the toe. Film (3) has a flat curve but the shoulder and toe areas show a more obvious transition than in Film 2.

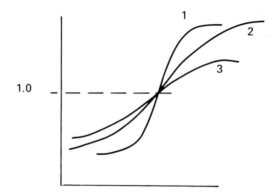

Figure 16. All three curves represent the same speed but different contrasts.

It can be stated that the shape of the curve tells the technologist two important film characteristics: contrast and latitude. Film contrast has already been defined as the ability of a film to record varying intensities of remnant photons. Film latitude is the same, but when the term latitude is used it specifically refers to how well the film can record varying photon intensities at the transition point of the curve where the shoulder and the toe meet the body.

Film Latitude

Film latitude is an important factor because valuable diagnostic information is often lost in these transition points. For example, when a radiograph is made of the chest, much of the lung field is in the upper

Figure 17. Film A represents a wide latitude (low contrast) film while film B represents a narrow latitude (high contrast) film. Actual H & D curves were made with these films; note that curve A takes a more gradual turn at the shoulder compared to curve B. By reviewing these radiographs it can be seen that film contrast plays an important role in the ultimate diagnostic image, since subject contrast can be altered by film contrast. The H & D curves were drawn to represent the contrast of the films; all other factors were held constant.

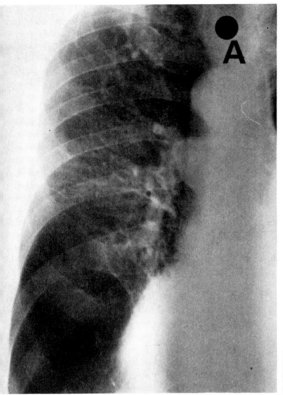

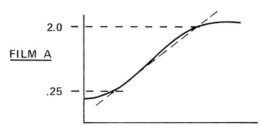

FILM A

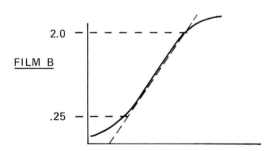

FILM B

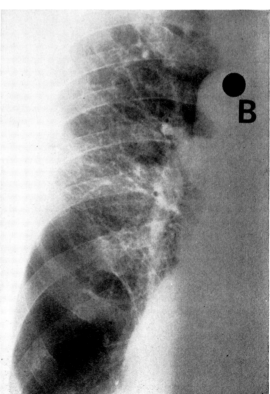

density region of the curve; if the film being used produces a very abrupt transition from body to shoulder, the film is known as a narrow latitude film. Because of the film's ability to make a quick transition at these points, some detail could be lost. However, a film with wide latitude characteristics would have little or no difficulty recording detail in the transition areas because of the gradual and smooth transition the film makes from the body to the shoulder or toe areas. Figure 17 (A and B) shows a radiograph of the same chest made with a narrow latitude film and a wide latitude film. If one is looking for detail at the densities at the lower end of the curve, a wide latitude film would again be more helpful because of its gradual transition characteristics from the body of the curve to the toe. The probability of seeing diagnostic information in this case is greater if a wide latitude film is used.

In short, it can be correctly stated that a wide latitude film is able to expand the useful range of diagnostic densities beyond what could be seen with a narrow latitude film, thus providing the viewer with more *patient information* (detail). It is generally true that wide latitude is desirable except possibly when examinations using contrast materials are performed or when subject contrast is especially low. It should be pointed out that film latitude and film contrast are dependent on one another to the extent that a high contrast film will almost always have a narrow latitude and a low contrast film will almost always have wide latitudes.

Film Contrast

Film contrast is the sensitivity of the film to various intensities of the remnant photons. Figure 5 shows a remnant beam emitted from an object has abrupt variations of intensities. In general, x-ray film can be manufactured to record these variations in three ways: to produce accumulations of silver quantities commensurate to the beam's intensities; to produce accumulations of silver that will in effect exaggerate these intensities; and to produce accumulation of silver that will result in an image which would deemphasize the beam's intensities.

Review the two gray scales in Figure 14. In doing so, we would see that the density differences in film (A) are more abrupt and obvious. As the densities this film produced are plotted on a chart, we note the body of the curve becomes very vertical, which is evidence that film is very sensitive to variations of intensity. Film (B), which was made using the same factors the gray scale produced, is more *moderate in gradiations* of densities from black to white; this is evidence that this film is not as sensitive to the intensities of the remnant beam. Thus, film (A) is known as a high contrast film and film (B) is known as a low contrast film. As will be pointed out in Chapter Two, all types of film have their place in radiography and one should be aware of the importance when making a choice. (Film contrast should compliment subject contrast.)

Determining Film Contrast from the H & D Curve

The term average gradient is used most commonly to determine radiographic film contrast. The average gradient for a film is shown in Figure 18. The average gradient is used because the true gradient or slope of all H & D curves change depending on which part of the curve you are viewing as it makes its tortuous route from the toe to the shoulder. Two horizontal lines are drawn covering a suitable diagnostic density range within 0.25^D and 2.0^D: These lines show the *average* gradient of diagnostic densities along the body of the curve. From these and with the formula shown below an actual film contrast value can be obtained.

$$\frac{D^1 - D^2}{Exp^1 - Exp^2} = \text{Average Gradient}$$

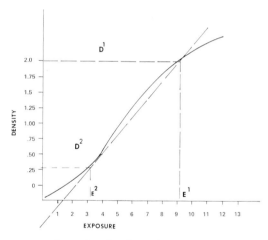

Figure 18. The average gradient for this hypothetical curve is 3. Actual film gradient values range from approximately 1.5 to 3.5. A film that has an average gradient over 1.0 will tend to exaggerate the differences between the various intensities of the remnant beam. Because of the low inherent subject contrast, film usually emphasizes rather than deemphasizes subject contrast.

From radiographs and curves shown in Figure 17, it is evident that one can choose from a wide range of film types. There are several terms used to describe the characteristic curves, but H & D and sensitometric curves are the most common. The body of the curve is referred to by other terms than those used in this text (two of these are straight line and gamma), however, these terms refer to actual angle or slope and not the average.

Base Plus Fog

If a film is processed without any type of exposure, it is not perfectly clear. This faint density, termed base plus fog or simply base fog, is caused by two major factors. First, the polyester material used in making the film's base is given a pale blue tint during manufacturing, to improve film contrast characteristics. Second, even though unexposed, a chemical reaction between the unexposed silver bromide crystals and the developing solution causes a low level of density. Base fog is always present in diagnostic film, but, under normal circumstances, it should never exceed 0.2^D. The presence of excessive base fog (over 0.2^D) causes a moderate to dramatic decrease in radiographic contrast, as well as an increase in radiographic density (see Fig. 19).

Figure 19

THREE MAJOR CAUSES OF INCREASED BASE FOG

1. IMPROPER FILM STORAGE
   - Storage Area Too Warm
   - Held Beyond Expiration Date
   - Unprotected from Fumes and Scatter Radiation
   - Excessive Background Radiation

2. IMPROPER SAFE LIGHT CONDITIONS
   - Too Many Lights
   - Too Large a Bulb Size
   - Scratched Filter
   - Safe Light Too Close to Work Area
   - Improperly Sealed Windows and Doors

3. IMPROPER DEVELOPMENT
   - Solution Temperature Too High
   - Solution Too Concentrated
   - Contaminated Developer Solution
   - Too Much Replenishment

CHAPTER TWO

RADIOGRAPHIC FILM

T HE NEED for an x-ray film was not to produce a visible image, because crude fluorescent crystals were already in use by 1895. However, the fluorescent image was very poor in detail and certainly not permanent (an image that could be easily stored for future reference was needed). The earliest types of x-ray film were actually glass plates which were coated with silver bromide crystals. These crystals changed chemically after being exposed and developed to yield a visible permanent image. One will occasionally hear the term "flat plate" being used, and this term recalls those days when the radiographic image was made of plate glass. One can easily imagine how difficult it must have been to handle these highly breakable plates.

A need for something more manageable was clear, and about 1924 the first film using a flexible base similar to what we know today was manufactured. The base was made up of a cellulose acetate material, and its usage was a truly revolutionary advance in medical radiography.

In this chapter, the basic composition of film will be discussed, and an effort will be made to relate how the components contribute to the desired result of a high quality radiographic image. The various physical and chemical processes that take place during the film's exposure to x-ray and processing sequences will also be introduced in this chapter.

FILM MANUFACTURING, AN ART

To classify the manufacturing of x-ray film as an art may at first seem presumptuous. There is no doubt that a high degree of technical information and scientific research weighs heavily in designing and manufacturing film. Yet, this raw scientific information has to be arranged and applied in such a way that the product will be of highest quality, much the way the composer uses the science of notes and harmonic chords to produce a symphony. The film manufacturers must work with the physical laws that govern the transfer of energy from the remnant x-ray beam to a latent image and eventually to a visible image. The laws of physics governing the production of a good radiographic image are common to all manufacturers. However, the ability of the manufacturer to work with these laws and their skill in doing so is truly an art.

DIAGNOSTIC X-RAY FILM COMPOSITION

Emulsion

Subcoating

Base

Subcoating

Protective Layer

Emulsion

Emulsion

Silver Bromide Crystals

Gelatin

Figure 20. Basic components of a typical double emulsion x-ray film.

Various Types of Film Composition

As complex as film composition can be, Figure 20 illustrates its basic parts. All x-ray film is similar in its basic design and composition. How-

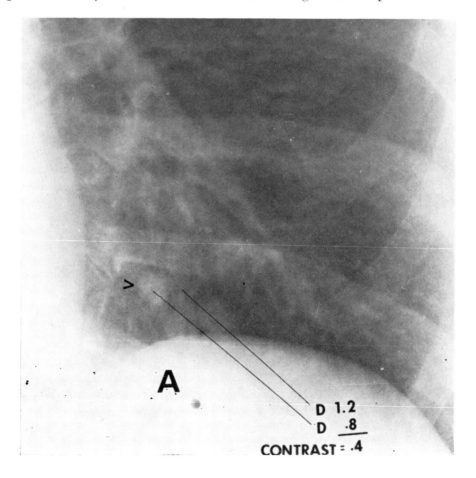

ever, there are some films that contain only a single emulsion and are used much less frequently in medical radiography as compared to double emulsion film. Today's needs for film are certainly more expansive than those of 1924 when almost any quality of permanent image was warmly greeted. It should be pointed out that x-ray film is also manufactured for industrial purposes. Our primary interest in this chapter will, of course, be aimed at the medical type. The most widely used type of diagnostic film is screen film. This film is made especially to be used with intensifying screens. Nonscreen film, also known as direct exposure film, is used much less often in recent years and is, of course, designed to be used with direct exposure only.

Radiographic film must produce an extremely high quality image, that is to say, it must produce an image that makes visible as much of the body part under examination as possible. As more and more body structures can be made visible radiographically, the higher the image quality

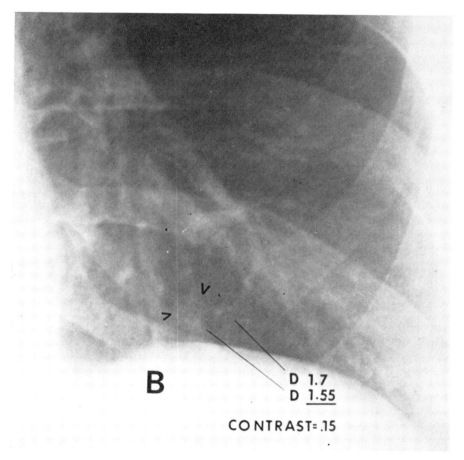

← Figure 21. *A* shows increase in visibility of detail as a result of proper contrast; *B* shows poor contrast and visibility of detail.

and the more valuable that particular film becomes. The types of diagnosis today's radiologists are trained to make are often so finite that only film which yields the best image possible should be used. Figure 21 shows some of these subtle but very important radiographic findings. One can easily appreciate how nothing but the best image should be used for diagnostic purposes. In a true sense, x-ray film equals the maximum that will ever be seen by the radiologist. During the author's research with major film manufacturers, it has become more evident that each component part of the film produced has been researched to the limits of reason and the substances used in manufacturing are of the highest quality available. The technologist should make every effort to position the patient properly and use the best combination of exposure factors possible since a high quality film cannot compensate for the selection of poor exposure factors.

The Film Base

The base is the support material of the x-ray film. Its primary purpose is to support the emulsion with sufficient firmness so that it can be handled easily. The emulsion goes through some important changes while the film is being transported through the various processing solutions, and here is where the film's base often meets its toughest test of quality. As mentioned earlier, the base was originally made of glass. Later, a plastic material (cellulose acetate) was used until the early 1960s when it was found that cellulose acetate caused some problems with film transport in automatic processors.

A polyester material is now used in its place. Modern x-ray film is sometimes referred to as safety film because of its resistance to fire. X-ray film can burn, however, but it requires much more heat and will burn much more slowly than the type that was used earlier.

Film Base Characteristics

The base must be fairly hard yet flexible; it must also be clear. (This does not mean totally transparent, but rather clear of any foreign particles that might detract from information held by the emulsion.) Light areas of the film appear as such because the emulsion has been dissolved away and light from the x-ray illuminator is transmitted easily to the observer. If the base was poorly made it might not transmit light properly or evenly and the light areas of the image would suffer. This could be especially important when viewing small structures of low film density such as lung markings in a radiograph of the chest. If a film is processed without being exposed to light or x-rays, all of the emulsion will be dissolved away by the fixer solution and you will see a bluish tint in the base. The purpose of this tint is to reduce the harsh light emitted by the illuminator. In short, a glare would be evident if the base was perfectly transparent and this would be very objectionable to the radiologist. By reducing the glare, the radiologist is better able to interpret the subtle density tones in the radiographic image. This might be similar to what happens as we walk down a street during a bright sunny day and try to see something located toward the sun. The glare and harsh light of the sun would make it quite difficult to see the object well. However, if you used a pair of sunglasses, the blue tint of the sunglasses would help reduce the harsh light and would increase the visibility of the object. Thus, the radiographic value of having a blue tint in the base is that it allows one to see the various tones of the radiograph more easily.

Base Thickness and Parallex Distortion

Base thickness has an effect on the sharpness of the radiographic image (see Fig. 22). You can see that each side of the film has its own separate image. The viewer, of course, looks at both sides simultaneously as the light from the view box transmits through the film. One can easily see that if the two images are not perfectly superimposed over each other a slight degree of blurring can result. Under normal conditions, this blurring is not excessive and is not a noticeable problem; however, one can see that the thickness of the base can have an effect on this type of image sharpness. As the base is made thicker, sharpness decreases. This type of blurring is commonly referred to as parallex distortion. Single-coated emulsion film does not possess this problem.

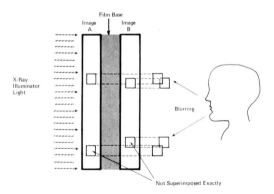

Figure 22. When *two different layers* of emulsion are used, the thickness of the base will determine the degree of parallex distortion.

A more practical problem that relates to base thickness is that regarding transport through an automatic processor. It can be seen that the tolerance in spacing between the transport rollers of the automatic processor is very important. Once set, the film must be able to pass between them with just enough pressure to assure transport yet not so tightly that excessive pressure would cause artifacts or a delay in transport (jamming). In general, the thickness of modern film bases is approximately .008 inches thick.

Base Plus Fog

It was earlier mentioned that the base had a slight blue tint, and in fact, this accounts for a low degree of film density when viewed. However, there is an additional density in the base that is caused by other factors besides the blue coloring. The base material is somewhat affected by the processing chemicals. During development, the base absorbs some developer solution causing a low level of chemical reaction which, in turn, causes a slight fogging effect. The third contributing factor to base plus fog (base fog) is low level radiation exposure to the emulsion of the film. The film is actually exposed to background radiation while in storage. Although this at first may seem to be inconsequential, considerable testing and troubleshooting throughout the country has shown this to be a more significant problem than originally thought. Many reports of so-called "bad film" have revealed the actual cause to be background radiation.

Base fog, then, is simply a low level density that can be detected on a film if it is processed without any exposure whatever. Quantitative standards have been established for acceptable base fog limits which should not exceed 0.2^D. If a reading is obtained greater than 0.2, radiographic quality could be in jeopardy. It should be remembered that very often important body structures to be seen are those of very discreet density variations: If they cannot be reproduced because of base fog, diagnostic value of the radiographic image is unnecessarily limited.

Silver Bromide Crystals

The silver bromide crystal is the heart of the radiographic image. It is what actually causes the density on the x-ray film. Manufacturing these crystals is very complex, and there is no purpose in describing it here. However, some characteristics of silver bromide crystals are important and these will be described here.

Crystal Size, Quantity, and Shape

One of the most striking things that come to mind is the extremely small size of the crystals used in producing x-ray film. For general purpose, screen type film, the silver bromide crystals are approximately 0.1 to 0.5 microns, and it is important to know that crystal size affects the quality of the image as shown in Figure 23. Although the size of these

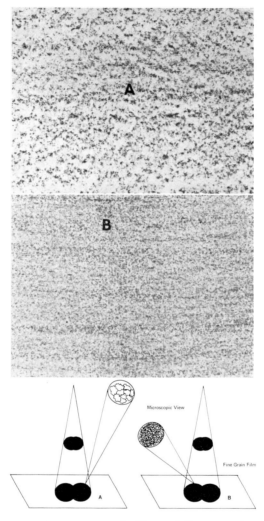

Figure 23. *A* represents a coarse grain film and *B* represents a fine grain film.

crystals has been enormously enlarged, the radiographic effect is representative of what actually occurs in a real silver bromide crystal. It can be seen quite easily that as larger crystals are used they individually cover a larger area. With such an increased area they are individually less able to duplicate body detail. Figure 23B illustrates an ideal situation as extremely small crystals are used. However, in Figure 23A one can see that these larger crystals influence greater areas of the image and decrease their ability to represent individual finite body structures. Crystal size has been increased to a point where one crystal represents too many body structures and cannot produce maximum detail. Since it is impossible for the same crystals to produce different densities, the film's ability to reproduce detail would decrease with larger crystals. With this in mind, one can begin to appreciate that an ideal situation is where each crystal influences only its miniscule area of the body part and can thus better represent the structure in detail. In other words, if crystals are produced beyond a certain size they will record neighboring structures as well as their own. When this occurs, radiographic detail dramatically decreases and produces an image that is commonly referred to as grainy.

Crystal Size and Radiographic Contrast

Crystal size can be varied by the manufacturer with a process known as digestion. It is very important that manufacturers control the size of the crystal because it affects the film's ability to produce contrast and density. As the size of the crystals vary with each other throughout the same emulsion, the film will tend to deemphasize intensities of the remnant radiation which, in turn, will produce a lower contrast image. It is the ability of the manufacturer to mix the various sized crystals throughout the film that produces various film contrast characteristics. Crystal size also affects the overall speed (sensitivity). As will be explained later in more detail, once a crystal has been exposed by the light of the intensifying screen or by direct x-ray exposure, it will change in composition and become black metallic silver via the developing process. It is important to understand that the more black metallic silver grains there are on the film after processing, the darker the overall image will be. If two crystals, one small and one large, are exposed equally, the larger crystal will indeed block more light emitted by the x-ray illuminator, giving that area of the film a dark appearance. A smaller crystal, of course, would allow more illuminator light to pass through the viewer and that area of the film would appear less dense. A film made with larger crystals will produce more overall blackness (density) than a film made with small crystals if both were exposed equally. In fact, changing crystal size is a common method used by film makers to produce film with various speed characteristics. The film with a fast speed will produce more density per exposure because its larger silver bromide crystals will intercept more x-ray photons, thus causing a larger black area in the film's emulsion.

The thickness with which silver bromide crystals are coated also strongly influences film speed for reasons that are outlined in Figure 24. It can be seen here that with equal exposure values, the film with more crystals (thicker emulsion) will absorb more photons, thus producing more black metallic silver during processing.

There is no typical shape of silver bromide crystals. A micrograph of a typical crystal used in manufacturing x-ray film would show that these crystals are irregularly shaped with many variations. The shape of the crystal has very little apparent effect on radiographic quality.

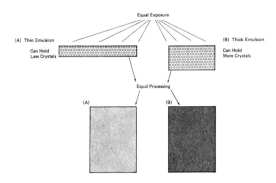

Figure 24.

Film Contrast and Latitude

Film contrast is influenced by using different crystal sizes in the film's emulsion. As the crystals become more varied in size, contrast will decrease; as the size of the individual crystals become more consistent throughout the emulsion, the film will have high contrast characteristics. Film latitude, as was already described, is the film's ability to record *diagnostic* densities toward the extreme light and dark density regions. It is generally held that a low contrast film will have a wide latitude characteristic and vice versa.

The Gelatin

The gelatin contained in the x-ray film's emulsion plays a very important part in the film's overall quality. Gelatin and silver bromide crystals are mixed to produce what is known as the emulsion. The mixing process is quite a delicate operation because any variation in consistency or in how evenly the emulsion is spread over the film's base will cause very obvious radiographic changes. If this *coating* process is not properly controlled it will affect radiographic contrast as well as density. The practical problem that this would cause to the technologist is that the same type of film would produce different densities and contrast values from one month to the next. With this kind of inconsistency, it would be very difficult to produce predictable radiographic results.

As refined and controlled a substance as gelatin is, it can simply be described as a clear gel which is refined very meticulously from calf's skin. Its properties, however, are much more important: (1) Gelatin must be perfectly transparent; (2) It must be able to hold the silver bromide crystals firmly in place, especially during processing; (3) Gelatin must be able to swell and contract during the processing cycles. One can imagine a radiographic image whose crystals have "slipped" out of position. Of course, this is not likely to happen, but it *does show any degree* of crystal shifting would be disastrous to the quality of the radiographic image. The task of holding the silver bromide crystals firmly in place is made considerably more difficult once the exposed film begins its route through an automatic processor. In addition, the gelatin must be able to resist the various chemicals with which it comes in contact during processing.

There is a moderate degree of friction against the film surface caused by the processor's rollers and, as noted above, it is during processing that the gelatin becomes most important in the radiographic image. As soon as the film is immersed in the developer solution, the gelatin begins to swell beyond its original thickness. During this expansion, the silver bromide crystals must be held in exactly their original position. The importance of the swelling lies in the fact that a situation must be created whereby the developer solution can easily seep into the depths of the emulsion to begin the developing action on those crystals located along the film's base. If the gelatin could not swell sufficiently during developing, underdevelopment would occur and the radiographic density and contrast would be decreased.

After this very important emulsion swelling period, the film is transported to the fixer and then into the wash where clean fresh water is used to "bathe" the gelatin of the residue chemicals from the developing and fixing cycles. The gelatin must undergo its last important change, shrinking and hardening, as the film is transported through the drier section of the processor. The film can then be stored for future reference.

The Effect of Double Film Coating

X-ray film can be manufactured with single or double coating; double coated film is the most common. The main reason is that intensifying screens are used in pairs as illustrated in Figure 25. It can be easily seen that a film with emulsion on both sides of its base would take advantage

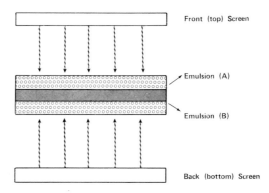

Figure 25. Double coating is essential to general screen radiography to make effective use of screen light emission from both screens.

of the light emitted by both screens. Two thinly coated emulsions are more practical than one thick single coating, because the light from the intensifying screens would not be able to penetrate the thick emulsion and expose the crystals lying against the film base. Also the developing solution would certainly have more difficulty in reaching the exposed crystals lying close to the base.

Film Storage

Film storage is a simple problem if one keeps in mind that the emulsion in x-ray film is sensitive to circumstances other than exposure by light or by the x-ray beam. The basic rule is to store film in a cool, dry area (50 to 65% humidity at a temperature from 40° to 70°). As the atmospheric conditions reach the upper limits of these regions, the shelf life* of x-ray film is reduced dramatically. Another factor in film storage besides the atmospheric conditions is that x-ray film is sensitive to various types of fumes and gases. Certain strong gases will produce a low level of ionization which will cause fogging. If film is stored beyond its expiration date, some very definite problems could result. The most likely would be decreased radiographic contrast and increased base fog.† The extent of these is directly related to how badly the film storage requirements were violated. It is not a good economic practice, however, to throw out film immediately upon the arrival of its expiration date. Upon the realization that a supply of film is beyond its expiration date, from a practical point of view a sample film can be pulled and tested for contrast and speed. This can be done by exposing a current and old film equally with a sensitometer and reading the base fog and a density at approximately 0.5^D. If both films produce equal densities the old film can probably be used.

LATENT IMAGE FORMATION

Although proper film composition is crucial to a good radiographic image, a process known as latent image formation is the mechanism by which the film's component parts work together with the exposure to produce the eventual visible image. The strange thing is that latent image formation process is only a theory, that is to say, it has not been totally proven. The reason for this lies in the infinitesimal size of the structures

---

* A period of time when something can be stored without danger of deterioration.

† Because there is already some density on the film due to base fog, the film will produce, depending on the degree of fogging, slightly more density than would otherwise be expected for that exposure value.

involved. In fact, the latent image itself cannot be detected by any means so far known.

In reality, there are many so-called "images." There is the radiographic image, the visible image, and the projected image, and all refer to slightly different aspects of radiography. In short, the latent image is the ionization of the exposed silver bromide crystals in the emulsion as *compared* with those crystals that have not been exposed and therefore are *not ionized.*

Before going into a detailed discussion of this important topic, it might be well to reflect for a moment on a more general level. Figure 26 shows that a structure can be made visible by making a number of black dots on a sheet of paper. Upon inspection of a routinely exposed and processed x-ray film, we should imagine that the various black and grey tones present are the result of accumulated or concentrated tiny spots of black silver. For example, if we closely inspect the composition of a newspaper picture we will begin to see that the image being viewed is made up of an accumulation of very tiny dots. You will also note that where the dots have become concentrated, the picture looks darker and the lighter areas are caused by a more sparse distribution of these dots. Thus, the radiographic image is nothing more than a series of random concentrations of tiny black metallic specks. As was noted earlier, the latent image is caused by the ionization of silver bromide crystals as a result of an exposure by x-rays or intensifying screen light. The greater the exposure, the more silver and bromide ions will be liberated within the crystal and will result in a greater latent image formation. In short, the latent image is the mixture or pattern of ionized and nonionized silver bromide grains as a result of the exposure.

ANATOMY OF A RADIOGRAPHIC IMAGE

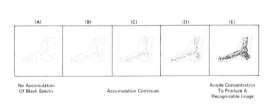

Figure 26. As the number of black metallic particles present in the exposed and processed film's emulsion increases, more body parts will become visible. However, *too many* black silver particles will decrease visibility due to excessive radiographic density and reduced contrast.

The Crystal Lattice

In order to more clearly understand the latent image, we will now introduce a structure commonly referred to as the crystal lattice. The lattice is a combination of atoms made of silver (+) ions and bromine (−) ions arranged in such a way that, when struck by an x-ray photon, the positive silver ions and negative bromine ions begin to move within the crystal in rather predictable patterns. The crystal lattice may be thought of as a single molecule of silver bromide.

In order to describe the process of latent image formation, we must gain some additional insight into the crystal of the film. The overall chemical composition of the film's crystal was described above and is illustrated in Figure 27. The lattice indicates that each correctly formed crystal has a specific and crucial arrangement of silver and bromine ions in addition to several small specks of sulfur compounds. The sulfur compounds are located in the outer edges of the lattice arrangement and are commonly known as sensitivity specks. Their purpose is to trap the free-floating, negative bromine ions that will be released when the crystal is ionized by absorption of light or x-ray photons. In a very general way, the lattice cube may be thought of as a closed environmental area in which these ions may roam after the exposure. When the exposure puts these negative ions into motion, the sensitivity specks trap them.

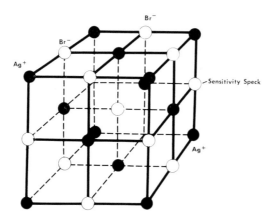

Figure 27. A schematic drawing of a silver bromide crystal is shown here before exposure.

The sensitivity speck is often referred to as a defect in the silver bromide crystal. The reason for this is that the crystal lattice provides a route by which the ions can travel after being liberated by the exposure. However, the sensitivity speck is an area of the crystal lattice that prevents easy movement of the negative bromine ions and in that sense are defects in the crystal. The defect has been described by Christensen, Curry III, and Nunnally. They compare the crystal lattice to a brick wall within which one row of improperly sized bricks were laid. The result of this incompatibility of structure is an increase of pressure on that defective row of bricks. Similarly, the crystal lattice has built into it an incompatibility in structure (the sensitivity speck) which will not allow the roaming negative bromine ions to pass by without entrapping them. With the above description of a typical silver bromide crystal, we may proceed with what actually causes the latent image.

We can begin the description of latent image formation by describing one random photon as it is emitted by the patient. Of course, many of these photons are not absorbed by the silver bromide crystal and no ionization or latent image formation results. However, those photons that do expose the crystal will cause ionization. Thus, the more photons of intensifying screen light or of x-rays there are to strike the crystal, the more photons absorption (by the crystal) takes place, and more latent images will result. When a photon is absorbed by the crystal, the negative bromine ions immediately begin to move about the lattice structure (see Fig. 28). The ions will continue to travel for some distance until they approach an area of increased chemical pressure caused by the sensitivity speck. The negative ion (see Fig. 29) causes the once neutral sensitivity speck to take on a negative charge. Simultaneously, the newly liberated negative ion may collide with other ions and release others from their

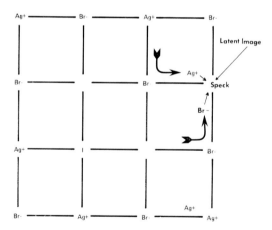

Figure 28. A schematic drawing of the same crystal after exposure. As a result of crystal ionization, silver and bromine ions are formed and begin to move about in the crystal lattice toward the sensitivity speck.

position in the crystal lattice as well. These additional bromine ions eventually accumulate at the sensitivity specks located throughout the silver bromide crystal. The positive ions are also released in the ionization process. Once the sensitivity speck traps a negative bromine ion, it acquires a negative charge and the more slowly moving positive silver ions are attracted to it. When the positive silver ions begin to accumulate at the sensitivity speck, a chemical change takes place resulting in the production of a piece of black metallic silver. The enlarged sensitivity speck once again has a neutral charge but soon begins to impede the flow of other negative bromine charges. It soon takes on the negative charge and begins to attract the positive silver ions, producing a larger piece of black metallic silver. This cycle continues until all of the negative ions in the crystal have been attracted to the sensitivity speck or until the film is placed in the fixer.

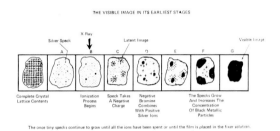

THE VISIBLE IMAGE IN ITS EARLIEST STAGES

The once tiny specks continue to grow until all the ions have been spent or until the film is placed in the fixer solution.

Figure 29.

The latent image is, in summary, formed by a process of ionization between silver bromide crystals of the emulsion. The once stable crystal lattice picks up energy from the incident photons as described and produces black metallic silver at the site of the sensitivity speck. A few last points should be made regarding the sensitivity speck before closing this discussion. (1) Without this chemical defect (sensitivity speck), the process of latent image formation could not occur. (2) There is usually more than one sensitivity speck in each crystal. (3) The number of photons striking the silver bromide crystal determines how many of the ions will be released and thus controls the extent to which the speck can grow. (4) The greater the accumulation of black metallic silver in the film's emulsion, the greater will be the film's overall radiographic density (see Fig. 30).

We must now direct our attention to transforming the latent image into a visible image, and this is accomplished by the reducing agents of the developer solution. Reducing agents, by definition, are substances that are able to give up electrons to another substance very easily. Actually, the overall effect of the developing solution is to simply act as a catalyst to the activities described above. It should be pointed out that the basic differences between latent image and the visible image is merely the size to which the sensitivity speck has grown as the result of the ionization process.

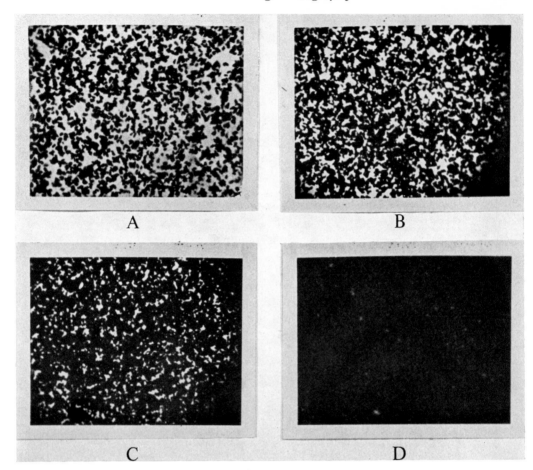

Figure 30. Four radiographs were exposed to various densities (*A* at 0.42, *B* at 0.65, *C* at 0.98, and *D* at 1.56), and tiny sections were magnified × 800 and photographed, in order to demonstrate that radiographic density is caused by the accumulation of black metallic silver grains in the emulsion. *Courtesy of* E. I. DuPont.

During development, the sensitivity speck becomes much larger and does so very quickly. For example, in a ninety-second processor, all of the silver and bromine ions are attracted to the sensitivity speck in twenty seconds. It is interesting to point out that a film could produce a visible image without the use of developer reducing agents—however, this would take an extremely long period of time, perhaps thousands of years. Thus, the developer only acts as a catalyst to the *natural activity* of the silver bromide crystal after the exposure.

Basically, what occurs is that the developer solution has an abundance of bromine ions to repeatedly give the sensitivity speck a negative charge, thereby attracting more quickly all of the free silver ions that are available. The sensitivity speck also acts as a doorway through which the reducing agents may enter with their abundance of negative bromine ions, as noted in Figure 31.

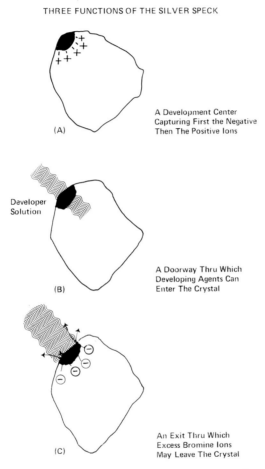

THREE FUNCTIONS OF THE SILVER SPECK

(A)

A Development Center
Capturing First the Negative
Then The Positive Ions

Developer
Solution

(B)

A Doorway Thru Which
Developing Agents Can
Enter The Crystal

(C)

An Exit Thru Which
Excess Bromine Ions
May Leave The Crystal

Figure 31. Without the presence of at least one sensitivity speck in a crystal, no latent image would be possible. No negative bromine ions would be trapped as a result of an exposure.

DEVELOPER AND FIXER SOLUTIONS

A textbook can be written on just the material involving the latent image, film manufacturing, and processing; the level of chemistry one needs to understand such a text is beyond the scope of our discussion. There are some general points that should be made to give a little insight into the composition of the x-ray processing solutions. Each manufacturer of developing solution has a slight variation in the chemical composition. However, the basic generic agents of developing solutions and fixing solutions are similar (see Fig. 32). The major difference in the composition of x-ray processing solutions is determined by whether or not they will be used manually or in automatic processors. Hand processing solutions are slightly different than those of automatic processing. The chemicals used in automatic processing have additional additives which prevent chemical fog, which is very likely to result from high processing temperatures. Additives that will aide in film transport are also included in the developing solution designed for automatic processing. This will be covered in more detail later.

Figure 32

GENERAL FUNCTION	CHEMICAL	SPECIAL FUNCTION	
	developer		
Reducing Agents	Phenidone	Quickly builds gray tones	Converts exposed grains to black metallic silver.
	Hydroquinone	Slowly builds black tones for contrast	
Activator	Sodium carbonate	Swells and softens the emulsion so that the reducing agents may work more effectively.	
Hardener	Glutaraldehyde	Controls emulsion swelling to allow better transport through automatic processor.	
Restrainer	Potassium bromide	Helps prevent reducing agents from causing chemical fog.	
Preservative	Sodium sulfite	Prevents rapid oxidation of the developing agents.	
Solvent	Water	Liquid for dissolving chemicals.	
	fixer		
Fixing	Ammonium thiosulfate	Clears away unexposed silver bromide crystals.	
Acidifier	Acetic or sulfuric acid	Stops and neutralizes developer activity.	
Hardener	Aluminum chloride or sulfide	Shrinks and hardens the emulsion.	
Preservative	Sodium sulfite	Maintains chemical balance of fixer.	
Solvent	Water	Liquid for dissolving chemicals.	

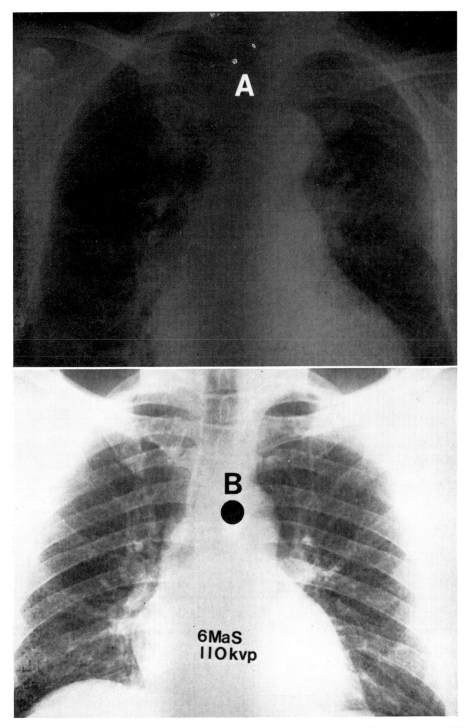

Figure 33. *A* shows decreased visibility of detail due to extreme chemical fog, while *B* shows a properly processed film.

Chemical Fog

Figure 33 shows the effect of severe chemical fog radiographically. Chemical fog, as you can see, increases density and reduces contrast substantially. Chemical fog results when reducing agents *invade* the *unexposed* silver bromide crystals. These crystals would ordinarily not be reduced and would be washed away from the surface of the film. The radiographic image, of course, depends solely on differences between one tone and another, which means that the white or lighter areas of the image are as important to maintain as are the black. If reducing agents invade the unexposed crystal (which should appear white on the film) the white areas would begin to diminish and darken slightly as a certain amount of black metallic silver is produced. Thus a buildup of density in these *inappropriate areas* gives rise to an overall grey flat look. Chemical fog is caused by reduction (see Fig. 34) of unexposed silver bromide crystals causing a decrease in radiographic contrast and an increase in radiographic density.

There are only a few things that can commonly cause reducing agents to attack and reduce unexposed crystals; they are (1) too high a developing solution temperature; (2) using a highly concentrated solution; (3) too long a developing time, and (4) contamination of solutions.

Figure 34.

COMMON CAUSES OF CHEMICAL FOG

1. ⋏ Developing Temperature
2. ⋏ Developing Time
3.   Chemical Contamination
4. ⋏ Replenishment
5.   Chemical Imbalance;
     –Weak Restrainer

Note: Chemical fog occurs when *unexposed* silver bromide grains are converted to black metallic silver.

The fixing solution has, by comparison, a rather sedentary role in film processing, and its chemical balance in general is not as delicate as that of the developer. However, a certain degree of control must be maintained for good processing. The basic purposes of the fixer are that it dissolve the unexposed crystals from the film's emulsion and harden the emulsion so that the film can be put into storage. In summary, it is the fixer that clears the film so the light areas of the film can be produced. It should be pointed out, further, that the fixer will dissolve the black metallic silver from the film, causing a bleaching effect *if* fixing time is extended for several hours. Thus, the fixer solution can reverse the effect of the reducing agent. Under normal conditions, once the film is placed in the fixer all developing activity ceases.

CHAPTER THREE

AUTOMATIC PROCESSING

INTRODUCTION

O NE OF THE most important pieces of equipment in a radiology department is a reliable processor. Over the past ten years automatic processing has come a long way in design and dependability. Proof of this
is in the total dependency all departments have placed over recent years
in automatic processing units. In this chapter, the fundamental design
and its functioning systems will be discussed with some emphasis on
troubleshooting, malfunctions, and breakdowns. It has been the author's
opinion that overall radiographic quality is not possible until there is at
least a general working knowledge regarding a processor's component
parts.

Figure 35 is a photograph of a conventional darkroom that was used
up until the late 1950s. With some imagination one can begin to see some
of the more obvious problems common to the manual method of x-ray

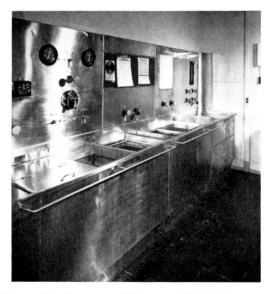

Figure 35. *Courtesy of* Eastman Kodak Company.

[47]

film processing. Each film had to be individually racked on metal frames and placed in various solution tanks. This became a problem when large quantities of film had to be handled at the same time. The "racked" films were placed in the developing tank for three to five minutes, then into the rinse and fixer tanks. In the meantime, the darkroom attendant's hands were wet and, before another batch of film could be put into the developing tank, had to be dried. Manual timers had to be set for each developing, fixing, and washing phase, and sometimes two different batches of films were placed in the same tank at different times. The darkroom attendant was often literally in solutions up to his elbows. In addition to all this, it was impossible for anyone to view the film for quality until at least eight to ten minutes had elapsed after the film was sent to the darkroom for processing. Needless to say, replenishing the solutions was a messy affair; in addition to all the other duties, the darkroom attendant had to maintain a fairly accurate log relative to the number of films processed so that he would know when the solutions needed to be replenished with fresh solution.

As a result of all this film handling and general activity, a lack of control occurred; coupled with long periods of time wasted waiting for film to progress through the various solution tanks, there was much interest in replacing this method with something more manageable and quicker. Thus the strong interest in automatic processing was to (1) increase department efficiency by making the finished radiographs available more quickly (hopefully to the extent where it would be practical for a technologist to keep a patient on the table until the film was viewed); (2) reduce the mess of wet darkroom floors and walls, a result of open developer fixer tanks evaporating into the room air; (3) reduce artifacts by limiting the number of times the film's delicate surface had to be handled; and (4) help stabilize radiograph quality.

Centralized Versus Dispersal Processing

Indeed the use of automatic processors has proliferated over the past fifteen years to the point where they are now taken for granted. Depending on the configuration of the department, automatic processors can be used in one of two basic ways: centralized and dispersal. Centralized processing is when one or two processors are centrally located in the department. The result of this is that very often technologists have to transport cassettes long distances to the darkroom. Also, a large backlog of cassettes to be processed is very common, resulting in long waiting times. The dispersal processing system is utilized when several processors are strategically located throughout the various sections of the department to serve just a few rooms. The result of this is reduced transport of the exposed cassettes through the halls, and because the processor is responsible for fewer radiograph rooms there is less waiting. This arrangement is generally considered to be more efficient.

Early Automatic Processors

The first automatic processor was installed about 1959. It measured approximately ten feet long, five feet high, and thirty inches wide. Figure 36 shows the relative size of the first Kodak M processor compared with the new Kodak M6A-N®. The M completely processed a film in seven minutes (dry to dry). This was less time than could be done in just the developing and fixing alone using the manual method.

With automatic processing the darkroom has taken on a new look and function. It has become much smaller and more pleasant to work in.

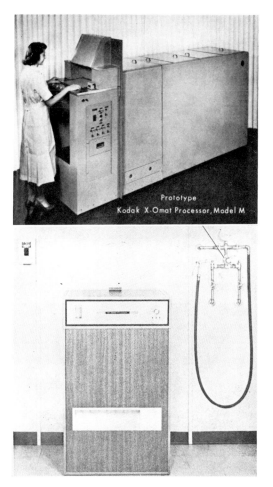

Figure 36. *Courtesy of* Eastman Kodak Company.

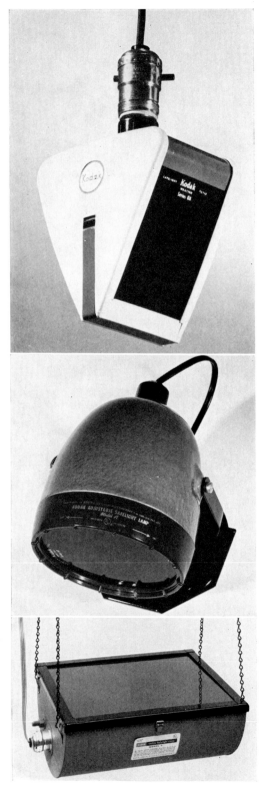

Figure 37. *Courtesy of* Eastman Kodak Company.

The prerequisites for a modern darkroom are much simpler by comparison. A floor drain is needed. A simple hot and cold water supply is connected to the now familiar mixing valve, and an appropriate arrangement of pass boxes (depending on whether the dispersal or centralized system is used) are installed. Sufficient counter space, 220 volts of electrical power, a film bin, and a good ventilation system are needed as well. There must be, of course, an ample supply of safe light fixtures. The types of safe light most commonly used are shown in Figure 37. It has a reddish lens and is known as 6-B wratten filter. It projects a reddish light to which x-ray film is not sensitive, thus causing no exposure on the final image if used properly. Other types of filters may be necessary depending on the film used. A wratten 2 filter is used for film sensitive to ultraviolet light. The term *safe light* instills a sense of false security, because if improperly used some light rays do escape to expose the film. Such an exposure to safe light is known as postexposure. Postexposure produces an unwanted increase in density and decreased radiographic contrast. A 10-watt bulb should be used and the fixture should be no closer to the film than two feet. Under these conditions, the film can be handled safely using the safe light for a period of no more than thirty seconds (or at three feet for sixty seconds). An indirect type of safe light fixture can also be mounted in the ceiling. Although more expensive, it often produces a much brighter light throughout the entire darkroom. Safe lighting should not be used at all with ceni film as well as other films with a *photographic* type of emulsion.

SOME IMPORTANT CONSIDERATIONS
FOR AUTOMATIC PROCESSING

As was pointed out earlier, manual processing was a terribly inefficient operation relative to space consumption, mess, and wasted time. Typically, a film had to be placed in the developer for an average of five minutes, rinsed for thirty seconds, fixed for ten more minutes, washed for at least thirty minutes, and dried by a variety of methods that could take approximately thirty minutes additional time. Thus the total time taken for this operation was approximately seventy-five minutes, or almost two hours. The chemicals and the film used were, of course, especially balanced and designed for such a slow system, which featured slow activity of the developing solution and relatively low solution temperatures that ranged between 68 and 75° Farenheit. The advent of automatic processing (dry to dry) systems, however, placed new demands on the developing and fixing solutions because of the new requirement for extremely short developing times and the use of developing temperatures of approximately 90 to 95° Farenheit.

Also with automatic processing, new demands had to be made of the film itself. Manufacturers had to produce a film that (1) could build a visible image very quickly; (2) would be able to be transported through a roller system without damage; and (3) had an emulsion able to resist relatively high developing temperatures without melting or accumulating chemical fog.

One of the important changes that was made in the film to be used with automatic processing was a reduction in the thickness of its emulsion. Figure 38 illustrates why this was done. Since the gelatin is not visible in the finished radiographic image, and because it inhibits the developer solution's progress to the exposed silver crystals, a reduction of its bulk made the silver bromide crystals more vulnerable to the processing solutions, and thus development could occur more quickly. Also, fewer silver bromide crystals were used in the emulsion. This might be some cause for concern since it is the silver that eventually produces the image we see, but careful calculations had been made regarding the overall quantity of silver that must be initially present in the emulsion to produce optimum results, and considerable care was taken by the manufacturers to stay well within the limits. The first important consideration regarding rapid processing is that a compatible film (thin emulsion) is used so that the developer solution can more readily penetrate through its bulk and

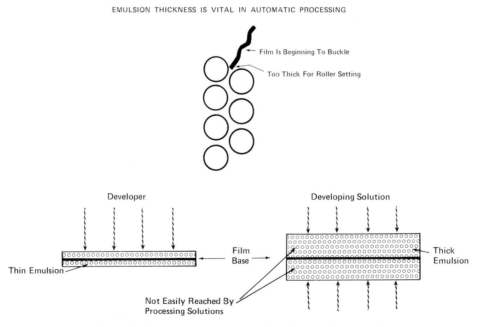

Figure 38. Emulsion thickness has not been reduced to the extent of detracting measurably from radiographic quality.

attack the exposed silver crystal. Also, of course, much care was taken in the design of the emulsion, to allow it to withstand the high developing temperatures of automatic processing so the gelatin would not liquify.

In summary, the primary changes in film composition were (1) to reduce the thickness of the emulsion (less gelatin primarily) and (2) to make the film's emulsion more resistant to higher developing temperatures. With regard to the processing solutions themselves, their composition had to be changed for several reasons: (1) a properly exposed radiographic film would otherwise be overdeveloped by the increased temperature and hyperactivity of the processing solution; (2) a more effective preservative had to be added to the solution to retard oxidation caused by high solution temperatures; and (3) hardening additives had to be added to the developer to prevent the film's emulsion from softening too much and gumming the processor's transport rollers.

MAJOR SYSTEMS IN AUTOMATIC PROCESSORS

The Transport System

In manual processing, the darkroom attendant moved film from one tank to another; with automatic processing an interesting series of rollers and gears do the work. In Figure 39, we can see a unit of rollers known as a rack. In the early M model they were so large a ceiling mounted crane was used to remove them from the processor for repair and cleaning. In Figure 40, we see the arrangement of racks and crossovers used in more modern automatic processors. The accompanying schematic illus-

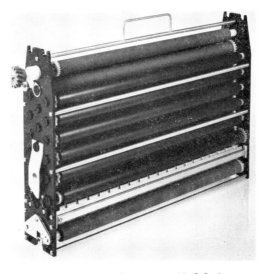

Figure 39. *Courtesy of* Eastman Kodak Company.

tration shows how the units are able to transport a film from the entrance
rollers to the bin of the processor.

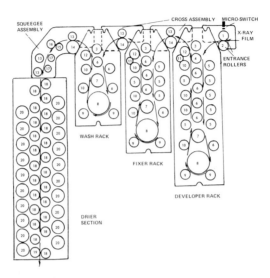

Figure 40. *Courtesy of* Eastman Kodak Company.

Thus the transport system's function is to move the film through the
various processing solutions and drying tubes without damage to the film's
surface. Another important characteristic of a processor's transport system
is that it must move the film at a very consistent and controlled rate of
speed. All other things being equal, the speed of the film moving through
a processor determines the developing, fixing, washing, and drying time.

The Margin of Error

With manual processing, developing time was so long that a thirty-
second error would not have had an especially damaging effect on the
film's image. By comparison, with automatic processing a five-second error
in developing time would cause a notable change. The automatic processor is much like a high powered racing car: It will go faster but will
tolerate very little errors in fine tuning. With automatic processing, the
total developing time, for example, is approximately twenty seconds. This
is certainly fast and a five second error (plus or minus) can cause a
20 percent variation in density.

In Figure 41, we can get a better idea of how all the individual rollers
function. A small motor turns a shaft which has "worm gears" set along its
length. In turn, each rack has a complementary set of rollers that fit firmly
into the worm gears of the main drive shaft. The rack also has a main
drive and its gear is made to fit a chain which turns all of the smaller

rollers of the rack. This general design is common to most automatic processors.

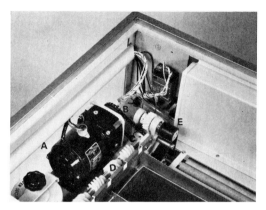

Figure 41. A—transport drive motor; B—chain drive to transport drive shaft; C— main drive shaft; D—worm gear; E—belt drive to dryer transport rollers. *Courtesy of Eastman Kodak Company.*

The Crossover Assembly

As the film begins its upward travel through the rack, there must be some way to eventually guide the film over into the next solution tank. Figure 40 shows how the transport system accomplishes this. The crossover, as you have probably already imagined, is simply a bridge that allows the film to cross from one tank into the other. You will also note a long metal plate which is located at all critical turning points. These devices, known as guide shoes, assure the film will maintain proper alignment between the next set of rollers.

As with most chemical reactions, some type of by-product is produced. In the case of processing x-ray film, *reaction particles* form on the film's surface as it is immersed in the developing solution; these are basically bromide and gelatin deposits. These reaction particles form tiny clumps on the surface of the film and, when allowed to accumulate in large numbers, act as a barrier to the developing solution (see Fig. 42). If a film had a coating of reaction particles on its surface, the developing solution would experience great difficulty in reaching the exposed silver bromide crystals in the film's emulsion and underdevelopment would occur. However, slight agitation of the film is sufficient to shake these reaction particles loose from the film. This agitation is accomplished by arranging the transport rollers in such a way as to cause a moderate bending of the film, as shown in Figure 44B.

In short, the transport system is an arrangement of racks placed in

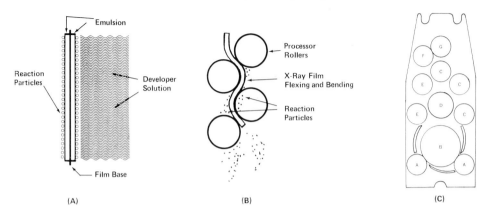

Figure 42. *A* shows an enlargement of film layers; *B* shows how the film is flexed back and forth to loosen the reaction particles; *C* shows the profile of an entire rack with the actual placement of various rollers.

each solution tank, crossovers, an assortment of gears, and an electric motor. It has two functions: (1) to move the film through each solution tank without causing artifacts and (2) to prevent reaction particles from accumulating on the film.

Artifacts Commonly Linked to Transport Problems

The most common artifact linked to transport problems is scratches. The direction in which the scratches run is important because it can help pinpoint the problem. Most, if not all, scratches caused by transport problems run the direction the film traveled through the processor. A dark scratch is common when the film is abrased after the exposure but before developing (see Fig. 43A). A light scratch usually occurs before exposure or the fixing or wash cycle (see Fig. 43B). If scratches (see Fig. 44) are noted approximately one and one-half inches apart running in the direction of film travel, they are usually caused by guide shoes that have come out of adjustment. Pi lines are white lines that run *across* the direction of film travel; they are frequently formed by new *processors* but this problem ceases shortly after installation.

Another type of artifact that causes plus density markings is known as pressure marks. It is important to know that x-ray film is very sensitive to pressure, especially after exposure. Any type of extraneous pressure against the emulsion, epecially during the processing, will cause the silver bromide crystals to overreact to the reducing agents. The result of this is an increase in density at the point of the pressure. Figure 45 illustrates this problem. With this in mind, one can imagine what might happen if the surface of the rollers is not smooth. Small but disturbing pressure (density) marks can be seen on the finished radiograph; they appear as faint, dark blotches. Keeping the rollers clean by scrubbing the crossovers daily and the deep racks weekly will help to reduce the possibility of pressure marks.

The Replenishment System

If a large number of paper sheets were continually dipped into a tank of colored water and the paper was so treated that it would have a neutralizing effect on the strength of the solution, the solution would eventually lose its color and potency. A similar situation occurs in the developing and fixing solution in automatic processing. As you know, the developer solution has a strong alkaline content, and the fixer has a strong acid content. As a steady stream of film is transported through these solutions in the automatic processor, the film's emulsion absorbs a certain amount of this liquid. Along with this simple absorption, an additional chemical reaction takes place in the film's emulsion, and soon the developing and fixing solutions tend to break down in strength. If this situation were allowed to continue, the resulting radiographic image would exhibit a marked decrease in contrast and density: The solution would simply become "exhausted." Figure 46 shows a radiograph process under this exhausted solution condition.

Built into all automatic processors is a replenishment system; its sole function is to maintain a predetermined level of chemical strength (activity) in the developer and fixer (Fig. 47 schematically shows its more important component parts). When a film is pushed between the two entrance rollers, they separate slightly to set a pair of delicate microswitches; these switches close an electrical circuit which energizes the replenishment motor which drives two pumps (one for the developer and one for the fixer solutions). As illustrated, each pump is connected to its perspective solution tank by plastic tubing. The fresh replenishment solution flows through the tubing past a flow gauge of the processor and into the appropriate tank. As you would expect, the flow of solution continues only while the entrance rollers engage the microswitches. With this system operating properly, the processor can then automatically compensate for the lost solution spent in developing each film. This, of course, stabilizes the chemical activity and strength of the developer and fixer solutions and prevents the possibility that they would become weakened and eventually exhausted. It is possible for a processor to pump too little or too much solution into the developer and fixing tanks, however.

Overreplenishment

Overreplenishment occurs when too much developer or fixing solution is pumped into the processing tank, thereby increasing the strength and activity of the solutions in excess of the prescribed limits. Typically, what

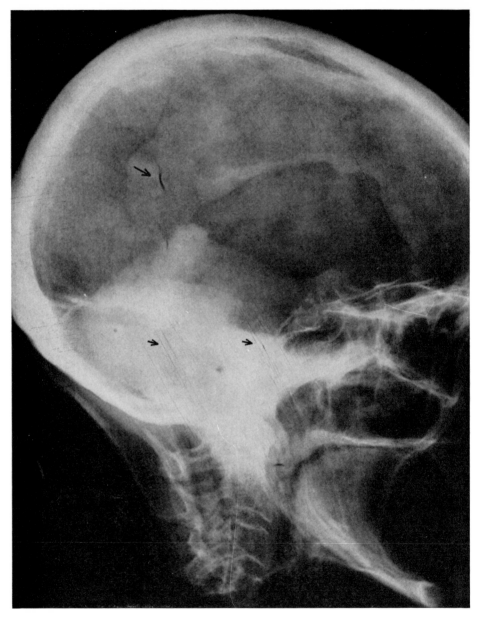

happens in this situation is that the developer solution becomes so active it indiscriminately begins to develop the unexposed silver bromide crystals in the film's emulsion. Thus, the unexposed silver bromide crystals are in a sense "forced fed" with reducing agents and begin to take on some density. Figure 48 illustrates how this would effect the image: the radiograph was properly exposed but processed in a developer solution that had been ovrreplenished. There is a sharp increase in density and a notable decrease in contrast. The film is too dense because the film was developed

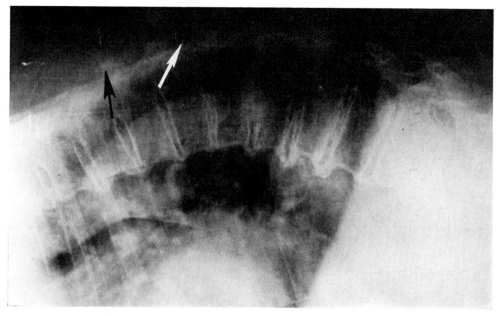

← Figure 43. In *A*, along with the black scratches, note the black "crescent" mark caused by the film being bent over a sharp edge such as a fingernail. *B* shows scratch lines that appear white, depending on when the scratch occurred.

Figure 44. As this unexposed film demonstrates, scratches may be caused by poorly adjusted guide shoes.

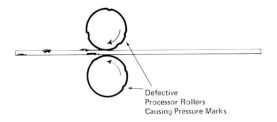

Defective
Processor Rollers
Causing Pressure Marks

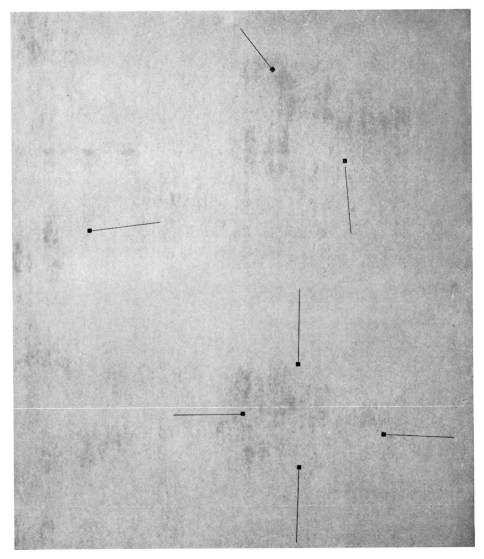

Figure 45. It is quite possible that these densities would appear more subtle than those shown here. The extent to which this occurs is dependent upon the degree of pressure by the rollers and in some cases film type. Certain film types are more sensitive to pressure.

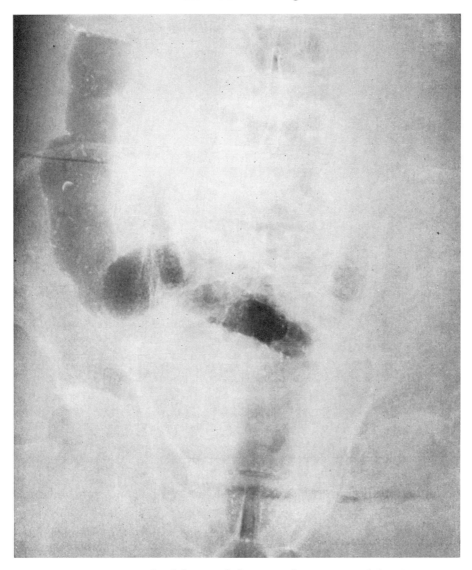

Figure 46. As a result of decreased density and contrast, visibility is poor.

beyond the correct level, and the contrast is reduced because the un-exposed crystals (which should represent the white areas) have taken on some density. Therefore the overall relationship between the black and white areas of the film is diminished. The most common causes for over-replenishment are (1) the flow rate is too high and too much solution from the replenishment tank; (2) the microswitches are set too closely and spontaneously engage the motor of the replenishing pump.

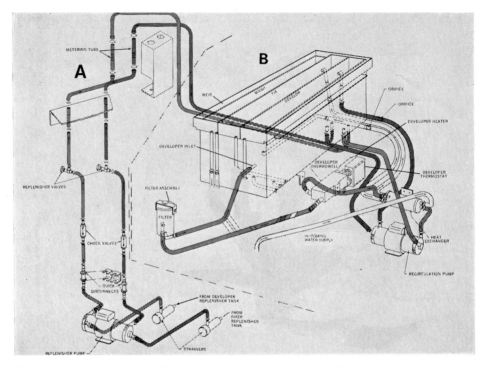

Figure 47. A composite of the recirculating system and the replenishment system. *Courtesy of* Eastman Kodak.

Underreplenishment

The result of an inactive or exhausted developer solution is decreased density and reduced contrast. Also, because the hardener additives in the developing solution are weak, the film's emulsion becomes soft and sticky, making transport difficult. With underreplenishment, not enough fresh solution is drawn into the processing tanks. Figure 46 shows a properly exposed radiograph processed in an exhausted developer solution. The strength of the developer chemicals are below the prescribed level to the extent that not enough silver bromide crystals have been reduced to black metallic silver particles, resulting in a marked decrease in density and contrast.

There are several causes for underreplenishment. One is that the micro-switches were "set" so loosely that they cannot close the circuit, even as the film passes through the entrance rollers. Secondly, the diaphragms on the pumps might be defective and unable to draw solution from the re-plenishment tanks. Third, the plastic tubing through which the solution flows to the processor from the large replenishment floor tanks could be pinched or blocked in some way. Fourth, an air pocket may have formed

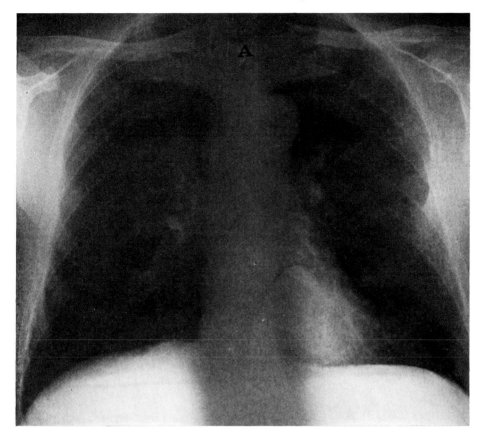

Figure 48. As a result of hyperactivity, developer reducing agents attack the unexposed silver bromide crystals and density begins to increase in what should be white or light areas of the film. Contrast decreases, producing an overall gray dense radiograph. A similar image can be obtained from excess scatter (S/S) reaching the film.

in the plastic tubing making it difficult for the pumps to draw the solution into the processing tank. Sometimes a pinhole, crack, or a poorly sealed connector in the tubing will allow such an air pocket to form.

The flow gauge can be used by the technologist to check what amount of solution is being pumped into the processor for each film put through the entrance rollers. Besides this, however, problems in transport or drying could be a clue to improper replenishment. First, it should be recalled that there is some hardener in the developer solution and certainly a great deal in the fixer solution. However, if replenishment is poor the hardener in the developer solution might be too weak and thus allow the emulsion to swell too much and become sticky and cause a jam. Also one might be suspicious of underreplenishment if an increase in abrasion marks are noted on the film.

There are many indicators to under– and overreplenishment. However, an alert technologist could prevent many of these problems by periodically looking at the processor's flow meters to see if the replenishment being pumped into the processor is the proper amount. Figure 49 shows the correct method for feeding film.

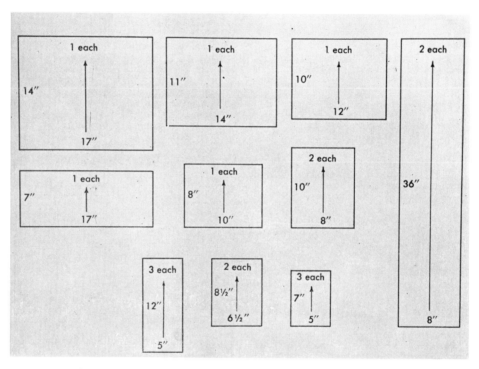

Figure 49. The correct method for feeding film into an automatic processor. If this is not done correctly, over development could result. *Courtesy of* Eastman Kodak Company.

Setting Replenishment Rates

The developer and fixer pumps can be adjusted to draw a specific amount of fluid into their respective processing tanks. Under normal working conditions, replenishment pumps work while the film is passing through the entrance rollers. If the flow valve is adjusted toward an open position, more solution would be carried into the processing tank and vice versa. Figure 50 shows such a flow gauge installed in a Kodak M6A-N Processor. The higher the metal balls rise with the solution during replenishment, the more solution is being pumped into the tanks. Figure 51 was supplied by the Eastman Kodak Company and outlines the correct flow rate for various conditions. You will note that the number of films one expects to process per day determines the prescribed flow rate.

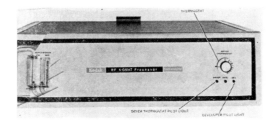

Figure 50. *Courtesy of* Eastman Kodak Company.

As the number of films processed per day increases, the replenishment rate decreases. Although this might seem contrary to logic, when solutions stand idle in a processor oxidation increases and breaks down and weakens the solutions. Thus with low volume processing, the tank must be slightly "overcharged" with fresh solution to compensate for the increased oxidation that takes place.

Figure 51. Correct replenishment rates. *Courtesy of* Eastman Kodak Company.

Average Number of Films Processed During 24 Hours of Processor Operation	Recommended Rates of Replenishment per 14-inch Length of Film Travel	
	Developer	Fixer
24	95 ml	135 ml
25–50	90 ml	135 ml
51–75	85 ml	135 ml
76–100	75 ml	135 ml
101–125	70 ml	120 ml
126–150	65 ml	120 ml
over 150	60 ml	100 ml

The Drying System

The drying system is designed to deliver hot air to the surface of the film after it has been adequately washed. It should be pointed out that the film is not considered totally processed until it has been dried. The drying system's major components consist of a heating element, a blower, a thermostat, and drying tubes. Figure 52 shows where these parts are located in the processor. The thermostat consistently monitors the air temperature being blown through the plastic tubing of the dryer section. If the air temperature goes below a prescribed level, the thermostat will close an electrical circuit, and the heater will automatically bring the air temperature to the required level.

Normal drying temperature is approximately 120 degrees Fahrenheit. Usually, there is little need to vary this range except possibly when a long run of roll type film is being processed when the temperature might be increased to 150 degrees. Drying temperature is certainly influenced by atmospheric humidity.

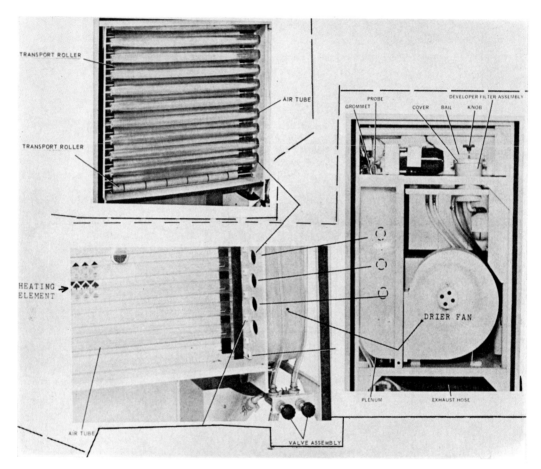

Figure 52. *Courtesy of* Eastman Kodak Company.

Drying Problems

Drying artifacts are not uncommon and are often indicators of problems that exist not in the drying system itself but rather with the strength of the developer and fixing solutions. If the replenishment system is under-replenishing the developer and fixer solutions, the film's emulsion might be too soft and unable to dry quickly enough in the dryer. Also, inadequate washing will often result in a greasy, shiny-looking film.

The Recirculating System

The recirculating system is possibly the most involved of the four major systems in the automatic processor. It has three basic functions:

(1) to filter out reaction particles and other chemical impurities in the developer solution and thereby help maintain its strength; (2) to agitate the developer solution so that chemical components will be equally dispersed throughout the processing tank; (3) to maintain and stabilize the temperature of the developing solution. The reader should recall the concept of time-temperature processing. It has also been pointed out that automatic processors do not allow a wide latitude for malfunctions before a deleterious effect on radiograph quality results and that maintaining temperature is a very important aspect of good quality processing. Figure 53 shows three radiographs that were equally exposed but processed at different developing temperatures. You will note the obvious density and contrast variation that ultimately result. For any given developer solution, as the temperature increases a condition known as chemical fog sets in. Chemical fog is the result of hyperactive solution or prolonged developing time. Chemical fog causes an increase in radiographic density and a notable decrease in radiographic contrast.

In Figure 47B, a schematic of the recirculating system is depicted. As the reaction particles fall from the film, a sludge accumulates in the developing tank. These reaction particles are eventually filtered out by a filter which is located in the recirculating system. The reader will also note the circulation pattern of both the fixer and developer solutions. The developer solution temperature is held constant by balancing it with the incoming cool water and the developer heater located in the heat exchanger. Optimal developing temperature is considered to be from 92 to 95° F. A developer thermostat (for the developer solution) is always monitoring the solution temperature as noted in the illustration. If the solution goes below a predetermined level, the thermostat will close an electrical circuit and the heater will begin to warm the solution to the desired level; once obtained, the thermostat will open the circuit and the heater will turn off until it is signaled by the thermostat once again that the solution temperature is too low. A small red light will brighten in the front of the processor panel when the developer heater is working. The developing solution passes through a device known as a heat exchanger, which is simply a heat conduction device. If, however, the developing temperature begins to rise too high, the heat exchanger could be used to lower the temperature to the desired level if the incoming water would be deliberately lowered by the technologist to perhaps 65° or 70°. As the cold water begins to pass through the heat exchanger, the metal casing cools down and the neighboring metal casing through which the developer solution flows would also begin to cool. In this manner the developing solution is refrigerated and could drop from 110° to 94° in approximately twenty minutes.

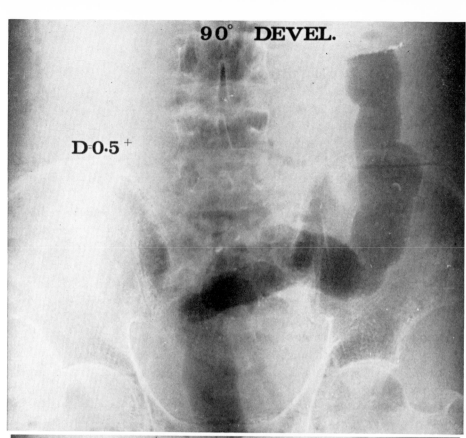

90° DEVEL.

D=0.5 +

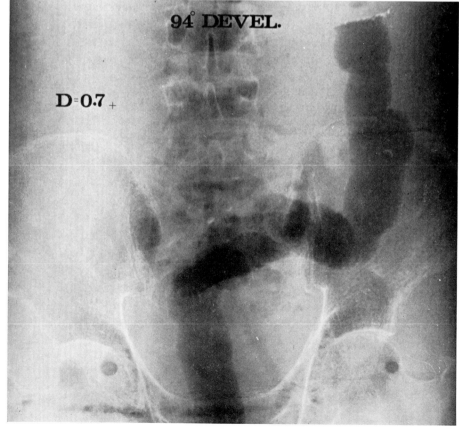

94° DEVEL.

D=0.7 +

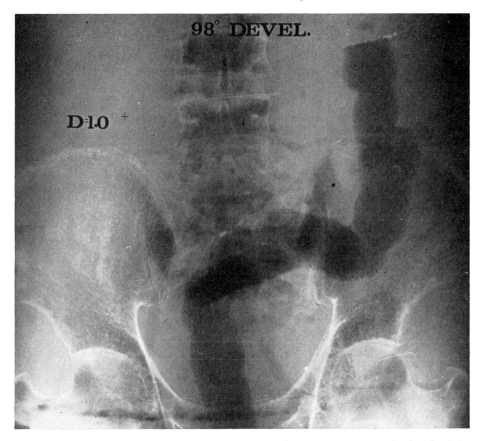

← Figure 53. Developer solution temperatures play an important role in obtaining maximum radiographic quality. As the temperature increases beyond its correct level, density increases and contrast decreases. Note the variations in film density ranging from 0.5^D to 1.0^D.

In short, the developer solution thermostat monitors the developer temperature and if necessary signals the heater to warm up the solutions. The cool incoming water is used to reduce the developer temperature if necessary and a small filter traps impurities so they will not accumulate in the developing solution and thus break down the strength (activity) of the solution. In general it is good practice to keep the incoming water temperature slightly lower than the desired developer temperature level. For example, the water temperature might be held at 86 to 88° and the developer thermostat set at 92°.

TROUBLESHOOTING PROCESSOR PROBLEMS

A great deal of effort has been expended in seminars dedicated to the sole purpose of uncovering some of the typical problems that can arise with automatic processing. The intent of this section is simply to point out some day-to-day problems and offer some suggestions that might help in finding the cause. Many have already been discussed. In the author's own experience, the following lists the most common problems, in order of frequency, and their corrections.

Trouble	Probable Cause	Correction
Dark films	Incoming water too hot	Adjust mixing valve
	Developing thermostat out of adjustment	Adjust downward
	Overreplenishing developer	Adjust downward, check microswitches
	Contamination (might have an ammonia smell)	Drain contaminated tank, clean thoroughly, and use fresh chemicals
	Light leak in darkroom	Repair
Light films, poor contrast	Poor replenishment	Adjust microswitches Repair leaking pump, broken pump or motor Check for air in lines Check for pinched lines
	Developer temperature	Adjust incoming water temperature Adjust thermostat Adjust defective thermostat
Films have a brownish look	Inadequate developer, replenisher	Adjust replenishment
Films have a milky appearance	Inadequate fixer replenishment	Adjust fixer flow rate
Films have a greasy appearance, often accompanied by a high contrast	Inadequate water supply	Turn on water or increase flow rate
	Wash tank might be empty	Fill tank
Jamming	Transport rollers not turning properly	Check gears and drive mechanism
	Poor replenishing rates	Adjust system
	Guide shoes out of adjustment	Adjust guide shoe
	Feed tray not properly aligned	Align
Scratches	Guide shoes not adjusted	Adjust shoes
	Raised or roughened areas of a transport roller	Replace roller
	Nicks in feed tray	Replace
Black, flaky marks	Accumulation of algae	Clean tank and roller Replace filters in developer and water
Increased fog	Old film	Eliminate
	Contamination of developer	Replace solutions
	Increased developer temperature	Adjust
	Overreplenishment	Adjust downward
	Fogged film	Replace

Explanation

Dark Films

Dark films are usually the result of overactive developer. Developer chemical activity raises with temperature. As explained earlier, developer solution temperature is somewhat dependent on the incoming water temperature via the heat exchanger. Lowering the water temperature may be the only necessary adjustment.

Occasionally, the thermostat itself will malfunction and will unnecessarily engage the developer heater. Adjusting the thermostat down will often correct the problem.

Overreplenishing could easily occur if the aforementioned microswitches go out of adjustment and engage the replenishing pumps too often. The pumps will continue to pump new solution into the tanks and eventually the reducing agents will become too strong.

Contamination of the developer tank with fixer can occur with only 3 to 4 ounces of fixer. Under these conditions, the tank and rack must be rinsed thoroughly, the old solution drained, and new solution be put in its place. When the developer solution becomes contaminated with fixer, a strong ammonia odor will result.

Light Films, Poor Contrast

Light films are usually caused by a developer solution with low chemical activity. This may be caused by simple oxidation or by developing too many films compared to the volume of fresh replenisher being pumped into the processing tank. Poor replenishment can be caused by a number of situations: (1) Microswitches not engaging the replenishment pump when film passes through the entrance rollers. A simple adjustment can correct this. (2) Faulty pump or motor. Here one might note leaking of solution from the diaphragms of the pump indicating the solution is escaping through the pump before it can reach the tanks. (3) Air in the replenishment lines. Air can be sucked into the lines through a tiny pin hole or a crack in the tubing or in a connector. Air in the lines will prevent the pump from making an adequate vacuum and little, if any, solution will move through the lines into the tank. One can usually see the air pocket in the tubing and with some imagination and manipulation of the lines it can be removed without dismantling the system in any way. The pump must be on during the attempt, however. (4) Pinched replenishment lines will prevent the solution from moving when the pump is pumping. (This is a very common situation.) To prevent this from happening, a two-inch plastic pipe may be purchased and used as a conduit through which all the replenishment lines are placed.

It is, of course, entirely possible that the developer temperature is too low. It was discussed earlier what happens to the reducing agents when the developer temperature is low. Low developer temperature could be the result of a defective developer heater. The thermostat could also be defective or simply set too low. In the latter case, an easy adjustment is all that is necessary. It is also a possibility that the incoming cold water pressure is too high and has overridden the hot, causing the developer temperature to drop via the heat exchanger.

Films Have a Brownish Look

Oxidation of the developer is usually responsible when a low density, low contrast, brownish image results on the film. Oxidation is when air mixes with solutions and eventually breaks down their potency.

To correct this problem, the developer tank should be drained, cleaned, and refilled with freshly mixed solutions. In addition, the replenishment system should be checked and adjusted so the problem will not recur. Often the problem involves a low volume processor and the most likely correction would be a very high flow rate setting (see Figure 51).

Films Have a Milky Appearance

It should be kept in mind that although the same electric motor is used to drive the replenishment pumps, there are two distinct replenishment lines and it is very possible the developer could be working well and the fixer poorly. Basically the same regimen described in the section on light films should be followed, placing attention on the fixing side.

Films Have a Greasy Appearance

The processed film must be washed thoroughly of all the developer and fixer solutions. The problem is usually very simply corrected by opening the water flow valve to attain a higher flow rate.

Jamming

If the reader can remember the drive mechanism, it will be recalled that each roller responsible for moving the film has a small set of gears attached. The gears of each roller mesh snuggly under normal conditions. With this arrangement, all the rollers turn at the same rate; however, if one of the nylon gears is stripped, the roller pauses. If the film reaches that roller while it is slipping, it could cause enough of a delay in transport to cause a jam.

On the other hand, the film's emulsion might become too sticky, which would cause the film to adhere to the roller. This condition would cause a temporary delay in transport sufficient to cause a jam as the following film catches up with the first. Occasionally, one can find a film completely wrapped around one of these rollers. Such a condition could be corrected by examining the replenishment system carefully and making the necessary adjustment. You will recall with poor replenishment the hardener in the developer and fixer solutions would not be very effective and the film would become too soft and sticky.

Finally the guide shoes must be set so that the film will pass between the rollers at crucial points along its route. This is a difficult problem to correct because it is important to find the one guide shoe that is out of adjustment.

Scratches

Although the film's emulsion is firmed by the hardener, it is still sensitive to deliberate abrasions. The guide shoes, if out of adjustment, will make white scratch marks one and one-half inches apart in the direction of film travel. A simple adjustment will usually correct this problem. Often, the shoes are set to turn the film too sharply causing unnecessary friction on the film surface resulting in scratches.

Raised or roughened areas of the transport rollers cause unnecessary friction on the film's surface as it passes between the rollers. This situation causes indiscriminate areas of abrasions. Some rollers may be sanded smooth, but soon after immersion in the solution, the roller will probably become defective in the same manner; replacement is the best initial recourse. Pi lines are common in new processors and disappear after a short break-in period.

Black, Flaky Marks

City water can be extremely dirty to the point where algae will grow and actually accumulate in the wash and developer tanks and on the racks. This condition will advance to the point where black flakes of algae will float in the water tank and eventually become "pressed" onto the surface of the film by the rollers. Nothing can be done except drain the tank, wash out the racks with hot water, and thoroughly clean the wash tank. In addition to this, a new filter should be put on the incoming water lines before the mixing valve. In areas with dirty water, filters should be replaced weekly. To help obviate this problem, it is sometimes recommended that the water tanks be allowed to drain over the evening hours. Algae filters and algae sticks should also be connected to the incoming water lines.

Increased Fog

The causes listed occur with equal frequency. Old film can certainly be eliminated by a conscientious method of inventory checks. Contamination rarely happens spontaneously. It often follows a jam when film, rack, and crossovers are pulled too carelessly, causing fixer to drip into the developer tank or vice versa. Keep in mind that because the processing tanks are small, only slight amounts of contaminants are needed to cause this problem. Increased developer activity will cause a situation where unexposed silver bromide crystals are "force fed" with reducing agents. One can easily imagine that the unexposed crystals are as crucial in producing light areas of the film (which in turn make up radiographic contrast) as the exposed crystals are important in blackness in the image. Obviously if the white areas of the film become gray through improper developing, optimal differences between the white and dark tones would be diminished, and reduced detail would result.

In summary, processing problems are often caused by poor quality checks and maintenance programs. In general, automatic processors are made for long service. Basically, student technologists are not expected to troubleshoot an automatic processor, yet a working knowledge of the major systems is important. There are, of course, many more problems that could arise, but those presented above are the more common and can often be corrected by the supervising technologist or a trained darkroom attendant.

ROUTINE MAINTENANCE

Although the processor can take care of itself in many ways, there are some points that should be followed. First, the deep racks should be cleaned with an abrasive material like Scotch Brite® weekly. The crossovers should be similarly cleaned daily to prevent reaction particles from excessive accumulation. The developer filter should be replaced monthly or every 5,000 films, and, if the water supply is dirty, the hot and cold water filters should be replaced weekly as well. The replenishment should be checked throughout the day. Some processors have a very convenient method of checking rates as was noted earlier regarding the Kodak M6A-N Processor. It was mentioned that the water tank should be drained each night to prevent the accumulation of algae. Most hospitals have a solution company that performs a monthly maintenance check. With this inspection, rollers, gears, guide shoes, lines, pumps, belts, etc. are checked for wear. Any part showing more than a moderate degree of wear should be replaced.

Sensitimetric Strips

A method of checking consistency of developer activity should be devised, since this directly relates to the appearance of the radiographic image. The author uses a method that involves the use of a sensitometer made by E. I. DuPont which sensitizes (exposes) an x-ray film to varying intensities of light so that a gray scale will result after processing. After the film is exposed with the sensitometer, it is developed and the developing temperature is recorded on the film. A densitometer is then used to read the densities on the gray scale at two predetermined points. The densitometer reads the tones of the densities and they are recorded.

The base fog is also read and under normal conditions the reading should not go beyond a density of 0.2. A base fog reading above this accepted level indicates a potential problem. Usually, however, it is a result of the developer temperature (which might be caused by an elevated incoming water temperature) or simply too much fresh replenishment solution being pumped into the processor's developing tank. It should be pointed out that an elevated base fog reading will certainly indicate the presence of chemical fog and possible malfunction.

CHAPTER FOUR

INTENSIFYING SCREENS

O NE CAN EASILY lose sight of the importance intensifying screens have on radiograph quality. In early radiography, screens, as we know them today, were simply not available. As a result of this, and because the type of film that had been used was much less sensitive to x-rays, exposure times were unbelievably long. An abdomen exposure would require several minutes and the exposure time for a hand or a wrist examination was perhaps thirty to sixty seconds. As demands for higher quality images were made during the early 1900s, methods of making faster exposure systems (film-screen combinations) were being tested. Also, the early pioneers of x-ray technology had to cope with x-ray generators that were not able to produce very penetrating rays or adequately high milliamperage values. It was clearly understood, however, that even with faster and more powerful x-ray equipment, other avenues had to be explored that would provide a faster exposure system. These early pioneers soon realized that Roentgen's discovery of x-rays was made with help of luminescent phosphors. Phosphors are substances that can give off light when they absorb certain electromagnetic wavelengths such as visible light, ultraviolet light, and x-rays. The color of light given off varies with the particular phosphor being excited. But generally the colors emitted by the phosphors used in radiography are green and blue and ultraviolet. Further experiments with these phosphors showed that perhaps luminescence (the process of phosphors giving off light) could be put to good use especially because the phosphor materials are more sensitive to the x-ray photons than to the film itself. This is because certain phosphors can absorb (capture) more radiation from a given exposure than x-ray film, and so phosphors will yield a greater response to an equal exposure. Figure 54 illustrates this point. With 500 x-ray photons, approximately 150 latent images will be produced compared to only five latent images when directly exposed. Thus, the phosphors will produce an effect that is thirty times greater for conventional fast screens (sixty for rare earth screens).

The color of light these phosphors produce for radiography is usually

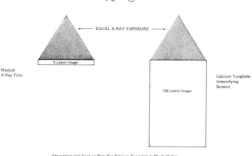

Figure 54. Exposure time, patient motion, and patient dose are decreased because of calcium tungstate's ability to absorb x-radiation as compared to the x-ray film. The actual ratio of "latent images" formed between a screen and nonscreen exposure is dependent on the speed of the screen being tested.

blue. Screen type x-ray film is, therefore, manufactured to be blue-sensitive, which is to say that a blue-sensitive film will respond better to blue light than it will to any other color. If the type of screen used gives off ultraviolet or another type of emission, one must be careful to use a compatible film, one that will respond well to that particular frequency. Thus the color of screen light used must be matched to the sensitivity of the particular type of film being used.

Another fact that inspired the use of screens is the deleterious effects of radiation to human tissue. Thus screens had another advantage, that of reduced exposure to patients. With the factor of reducing exposure time, and the added advantage of decreasing patient exposure, research on intensifying screens continued in earnest. We will see later to what point these advantages extend when modern intensifying screens are used. In summary, one might say the purpose of using intensifying screens is to reduce patient exposure and patient motion through more efficient absorption of x-rays. Screen radiography is possible because manufacturers can produce x-ray film that is more sensitive to the screen's emitted light than to the remnant x-ray photons. There is one important disadvantage with using screens, however, and although it will be discussed in some detail later, it must be noted at this point that screens greatly decrease radiographic sharpness.

GENERAL CONSTRUCTION

The gross anatomy of an intensifying screen is quite easy to comprehend. Figure 55 illustrates a cross-sectional view of a typical intensifying screen.

The Backing

The purpose of the backing is to act as a rigid support for the phosphor materials spread upon it. Originally, the backing was made of a card-

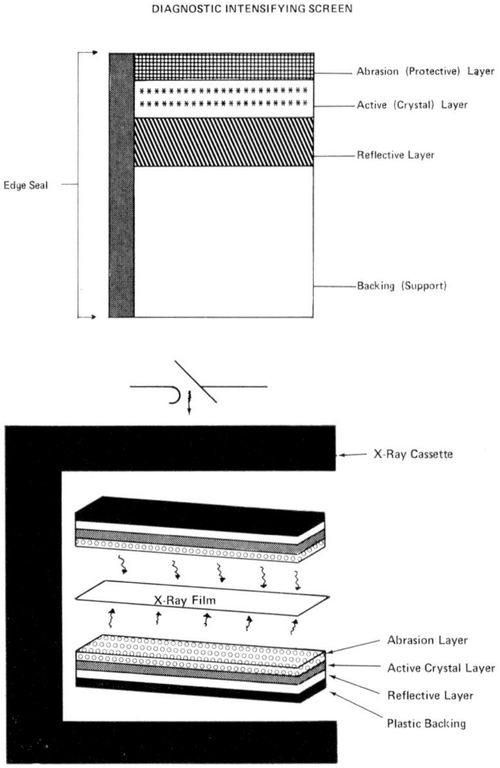

DIAGNOSTIC INTENSIFYING SCREEN

Abrasion (Protective) Layer
Active (Crystal) Layer
Reflective Layer
Edge Seal
Backing (Support)

X-Ray Cassette

X-Ray Film

Abrasion Layer
Active Crystal Layer
Reflective Layer
Plastic Backing

Figure 55. Although there is some variation between manufacturers, *A* is representative of most screens. *B* depicts a pair of screens positioned in a cassette.

board of high quality, but today a plastic material has become popular among some manufacturers and technologists. It is very important that screens and film surfaces make absolute contact or image sharpness will be substantially reduced. In order to assure good contact, the screens must be perfectly smooth and flat. With this point in mind, cardboard could be a disadvantage because as atmospheric humidity increases and decreases, a cardboard backing could expand and then contract. These changes would reduce film screen contact and decreased image sharpness can result. In contrast to this, plastic backing is not affected by moisture in the air and thus more consistent contact is likely to result.

The Reflective Layer

The reflective layer is the next component in the construction of a typical intensifying screen. As shown in Figure 56, its function is to reflect or bounce back light that has been produced by the phosphors. This has a direct effect on how many light rays will strike the film and be absorbed into the film's emulsion. Obviously the more light rays that are absorbed by the film, the more black silver crystals will be present in the visible image which would produce darker radiographic images.

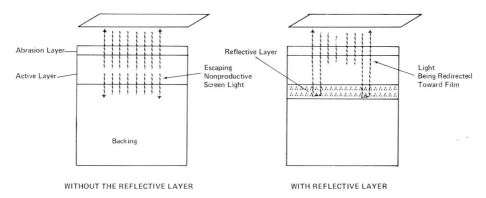

WITHOUT THE REFLECTIVE LAYER   WITH REFLECTIVE LAYER

Figure 56. The reflective layer is one of the primary factors controlling overall screen speed—the efficiency with which it can bounce escaping screen light back to the film.

You have already come to realize that it is the light from the intensifying screen that exposes the film and not the x-ray photons themselves. In fact, depending on the screens, only 5 percent or less of the density seen is caused by x-rays directly exposing the film. Figure 57 illustrates the concept that light is emitted by the photons in all directions similar to a lightbulb; if the stray light rays (green or blue) can be captured and redirected back, the film will experience a greater exposure. This is, however, accompanied by decreased sharpness. One can correctly say that, as

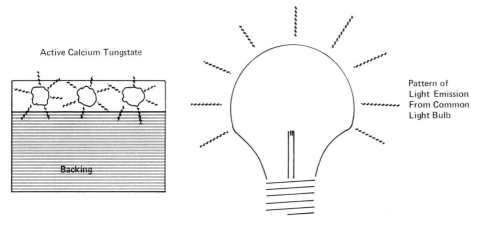

Figure 57. The root cause of screen unsharpness is the pattern of emission of the crystal. If the light from each crystal would travel in vertical direct pattern toward the film, screen unsharpness would be greatly improved.

the reflective layer becomes more efficient, image sharpness decreases but the exposure system increases in speed.

The Active Layer

The active layer is the heart of the intensifying screen. It has two components, the phosphor itself and the suspension material. The phosphor most commonly used is calcium tungstate. In the past, a phosphor known as barium lead sulfate was more efficient at absorbing x-rays and thus emitted more light. More recently, calcium tungstate phosphors were further developed and have improved to where their absorbing abilities are greater than barium lead sulfate. The active layer is approximately 4 to 6 $\times$ 10^{-3} of an inch thick, depending on the speed of the screen.

The suspension material that surrounds each calcium tungstate crystal and holds it in place is made of a plastic substance, thus its primary function is to suspend each crystal in place. Later we will see how these elements of the active layer can influence the quality of the radiographic image.

The Edge Seal

By reviewing the cross section noted above, it might be possible to imagine the radiographic effect if these components would begin to separate. The result in decreased sharpness would surely be great. This would most likely occur if moisture in the air would settle between the components and cause buckling and separation. To prevent this from happening, a sealing agent is used to cover the edges of a screen sandwich. Often, technologists will use too much liquid when cleaning screens—the edge seal will prevent excessive moisture from seeping between the screen's various layers unless a small crack is present in the edge seal (penetrating moisture could inevitably damage the entire intensifying screen).

THE PROCESS OF LIGHT EMISSION

Light emission is a phenomenon in which x-rays are absorbed by the phosphor crystals and react by emitting light rays. In the simplest terms, it is a process of energy conversion. A high frequency energy beam is absorbed by a substance with a relatively high atomic number (calcium tungstate) and in turn a lower energy of visible light is produced. Within reasonable limits, there are two types of intensifying screen, light emission processes: phosphorescence and fluorescence. Each gives off a visible light but there are slight yet important differences between the two, and there is usually a color distinction in the emitted light. Fluorescence, the more common of the two, is the type of light emission that occurs in diagnostic cassettes, is usually a light blue, and is emitted only while the fluorescent crystal is being excited (irradiated) by the x-rays. With phosphorescence, the emission, usually yellowish, continues after the x-rays have stopped irradiating the phosphorescent crystal. Fluorescent crystals glow only while being irradiated, and phosphorescent crystals can continue to give off light after the exposure has terminated (also known as after glow or screen lag).

Fluorescence

Fluorescence is a process in which a phosphor becomes ionized by x-ray photons and gives off light. The atoms of these materials contain broadened outer orbits that can be thought of as bands. Although much wider, these bands are actually orbits in which electrons are moving about. Figure 58 shows how the outer bands contain three different zones, each having a slightly different energy. A detailed discussion of the physics involved is not necessary here. Suffice it to say that such bands do exist, and their presence is an important characteristic of the fluorescent material. It should be understood that the inner orbits are confined to specific energies. It is only the outer orbits of these materials that widen and contain bands.

The various zones of the outer orbit are known as the filled zone, the trapped zone, and the conduction band. We can now begin a brief ex-

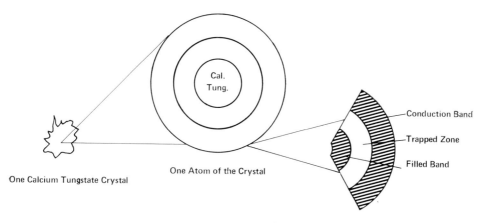

One Calcium Tungstate Crystal

One Atom of the Crystal

Conduction Band

Trapped Zone

Filled Band

Three Areas of the Outer Orbit

VALENCE BAND

Figure 58. Without these lower energy valence bands, calcium tungstate crystals would have no practical value in diagnostic radiography.

planation into the mechanics of screen light emission. In Figure 59 we see an entering x-ray photon has evacuated an electron from an area of the filled band. The entire orbit becomes very unstable and attempts to improve the situation by drawing on an electron from the trapped zone. As the trapped electron moves to satisfy the vacancy, which is in a lower energy level of the orbit, the trapped electron gives up its excessive energy so it will be compatible with the energy of its new location. This "excess" energy is seen by us in the form of green or blue light and goes on to expose the film.

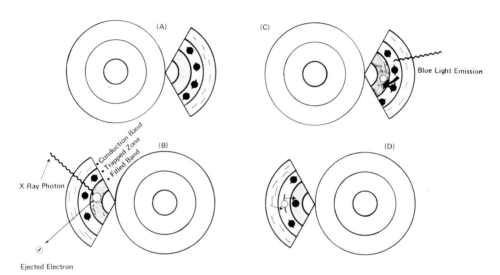

Figure 59. Screens produce light photons because of an ionization process. A, a stable atom of calcium tungstate. B shows an incident x-ray photon striking the atom's outer bands, causing a vacancy in the filled band, and resulting in the entire atom becoming unstable; in an attempt to become stable once again, one of the "trapped" electrons is pulled to fill the vacancy. In C the electron transfers to a lower energy band and must give up the excess energy to "fit" comfortably in the filled band; the excess energy given off is often the frequency of blue light and goes on to expose the film. In D the vacancy created in the trapped zone is filled by an electron from the conduction zone.

The amount of light emitted by a screen is primarily dependent upon (1) inherent ability of the crystals to absorb the x-ray photons, (2) the thickness of the active layer, and (3) the efficiency of the reflective layer. This process of light emission is caused by vacancies forming in the various bands of the outer orbit. As might be expected, there is a total reshuffling of the electrons located in this area as they begin to fill each other's vacancies. Also, with each reshuffling more light is emitted. This process goes on *only* as long as the exposure continues: Upon termination of the exposure, the ionization process and resulting light emission process cease immediately with fluorescent crystals.

Phosphorescence

Phosphorescent phosphors are very similar to fluorescent materials in general. However, the electrons are considerably slower in filling the vacancies created by the incident x-ray photons. In these crystals, the electrons in the trapped zone often do not have the total amount of energy needed to move directly into the vacancy in the filled band. During an x-ray exposure, the "trapped" electron travels to the conduction band where it gains additional energy to pass through the trapped zone and continue on to satisfy the vacancy in the filled band. It is possible, however, that an electron may not have sufficient energy to pass through the trapped zone even after it was somewhat revitalized by the conduction band. In this instance, the electron has to make several such trips to gain sufficient energy to pass through the bindings of the trapped zone. The procrastination or inability of the electron to immediately satisfy the vacancy in the filled band causes a continuation in the light emission process of the phosphorescent materials to the extent that they will continue to give off light after the exposure has terminated.

Phosphorescent materials are not often used in radiography today. They were, however, very popular up until the late 1950s and early 1960s when they were used by manufacturers to make fluoroscopic screens. Fluoroscopic screens were made with a phosphorescent material known as zinc cadmium sulphide. Since the brightness of the image produced was insufficient to satisfy current demands, an entirely new fluortechnology involving image intensifiers has evolved.

In summary, fluorescence and phosphorescence are light emission processes that are different in the color of light they emit, and whether or not they continue to produce light after the termination of the exposure. The light emission process is caused by phosphors absorbing x-ray photons and a resulting ionization process in which excess quantities of low energy emission (visible light rays) are emitted to expose the film.

Other Important Crystal Characteristics

It was thought by some that crystals themselves lost their light emission abilities with prolonged use. If the actual process of light emission described above is recalled, it can be seen quite easily that as long as there is an ample supply of electrons and vacancies, ionization and light emission will continue without change. Actually, the calcium tungstate crystals are quite stable (they can retain their electrons) and will produce equal light emission for hundreds of years of exposures.

Intensifying screen crystals have no particular shape and can vary considerably in both size and shape. With respect to size, however, most crystals used range from 4 to 8 microns, depending on screen speed. As crystal size increases, the amount of light it produces will increase when a similar exposure is used. Clearly, larger crystals will produce more light because they contain more atoms to become ionized and also will intercept more remnant x-ray photons than a smaller crystal would.

CLASSIFICATION OF SCREENS

The discussion up to this point has been concerned with a "typical" crystal and screen. Manufacturers can introduce certain chemical additives into the standard calcium tungstate crystal to slightly alter its emission characteristics. Other changes in the overall makeup of the screen can yield still further light emission differences. As a result, conventional intensifying screens can be categorized into three general groups based on their light producing efficiency. These are detailed (or slow), medium, and fast. Two of these types, exposed equally as shown in Figure 60, would yield strikingly different results. The screen that produced the darkest image would be known as a fast screen because it obviously produced much more light than the other two. By using a fast screen, the technologist can afford to reduce the exposure time by one-half and still maintain a comparable diagnostic image compared to medium speed.

The term *intensification factor* has important bearing because it tells the technologist to what extent a particular screen will intensify or amplify the x-ray exposure. Manufacturers can produce screens to amplify the beam by a certain factor. For example, if a medium speed screen was exposed using 100, Ma, ½ second, at 70 KvP, a certain density, such as 1^D, might be produced on the film. If a fast screen is chosen and the same exposure factors were used, the result in density would be doubled, equal to 2^D.

The significance of the intensification factor comes into play when new screens have been purchased for a department and new techniques have to be written or when the technologist knows he is about to use a faster or slower screen than was previously used. Generally it is unwise for a department to have more than one speed of screen available for routine diagnostic studies because of the changes in density that are bound to result in exposure errors. To find the extent to which a given screen can amplify the beam (the intensification factor), the exposure value needed to produce a given radiographic density with screens is

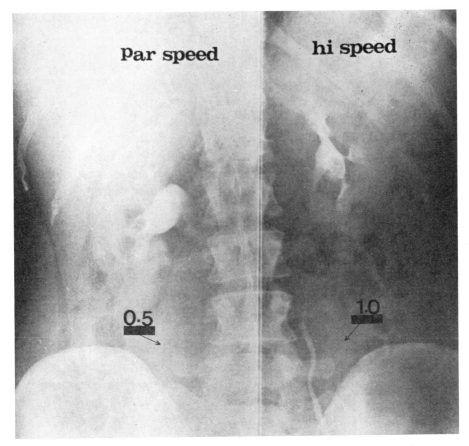

Figure 60. The variation in film density between fast and medium speed screens.

divided into the exposure value needed to produce the same density without screens.

$$\text{Exposure:} \quad \frac{(\text{MaS}) \text{ exposure without screen}}{(\text{MaS}) \text{ exposure with screen}} = \text{I.F. factor}$$

If a situation arises where 200 Ma, ½ second, at 70 KvP is used non-screen to produce a density of 1.0, screens at 200 Ma, ¼₀ second, at 70 KvP would yield a density of 1.0. With the formula above it can be found that the intensification factor for that particular screen is 20. The manner in which this information can be put to practical use will be thoroughly discussed in Chapter Eleven. The emphasis now will be placed on the concept that each category of screen has its own intensification factor and that I.F. tells the technologist the extent to which a particular screen will amplify the beam's effect on the film to produce the desired density. In screens with high I.F. factors, only about 5 to 6 percent of the remnant x-ray photons are put to use.

The Practicality of Having Different I.F.

In general, slow, medium, and fast screens account for a range of I.F. from 30 to 60 respectively. It has been pointed out that with conventional screens, detail decreases as faster screens are used. Slow screens are used for certain examinations simply because of the superior radiographic sharpness they provide. An example of this is the increased use of detail (slow) screens for extremity and, in some cases, mammographic work. Figure 63 compares the detail obtained when using fast and slow screens.

There are times when extreme detail can be realistically compromised somewhat in order to obtain a lower patient dose or to prevent patient motion. In such cases a faster screen is used because it can amplify the effect of the beam substantially over the slow screens. Examinations such as these might include pelivemetry and pediatric work. Examples for reducing patient motion include emergency work, portable work, and special procedures when very fast exposures must be made using automatic film changers. Also, many emergency patients are not able to hold still long enough to make a good exposure. Special procedures often require the run of rapid sequence films. Fast screens help considerably to make the exposure time as short as possible so more frames (exposures) can be taken while the contrast material is moving through the vascular system. Also there is a great advantage in special work in that fast screens reduce the heat load substantially on the x-ray tube. Between the two extremes of slow and fast screens, there is, of course, the medium speed screen which is in the view of many radiologists and technologists an adequate compromise between the advantages and disadvantages of slow and fast types. From this discussion it can be seen that there is a practical application for each group of screen speeds, and the proper selection is a matter of making an appropriate and realistic compromise between speed, patient dose, and sharp detail. Many more radiology departments are equipped with fast speed screens today than just a few years ago. The reason for this is that manufacturers have been able to produce improved detail characteristics of faster screens through constant research and product development.

HOW DO SCREENS AFFECT THE RADIOGRAPHIC IMAGE?

Contrast and Density

An image must possess only three things to be of high quality, but all three must be present: (1) sufficient contrast; (2) sufficient density;

and (3) sharply defined structures. The importance of screens in obtaining a high quality image cannot be overly emphasized, because they have a very pronounced effect on all three. The effect that screens have on radiographic contrast is important as well. Figure 61 shows two radiographs of the same body part. The exposure values were correctly adjusted so that density could be compared. Film B was exposed with a par speed screen and film A was exposed without any screens but with the same technique. Exposure for C was increased approximately forty-six times to produce a similar density to the screen film. Note the variation in contrast from B to C.

It should be clear by now that the light emitted by the screen is for the most part totally responsible for the diagnostic image. To illustrate this another way, two sheets of paper were fitted over one half of the screen so that the film would receive no light from the phosphors. The other half of the film was, of course, able to receive blue screen light. By viewing Figure 62 one can see the extent to which the unassisted x-ray exposure affects the film.

The reason why contrast is affected when using intensifying screens is not totally understood. It should be pointed out that radiographic contrast does not appear to change between the various speeds of screens but only in the initial nonscreen to screen conversion.

Screen Sharpness

With an understanding of the profound effect screens have on radiographic contrast and density, another interesting aspect of screen radiography may be discussed. It is vital that the structures radiographed be sharply delineated in the image. With all the advantages screens offer in radiography, they have an important disadvantage as they cause unsharpness. Whenever screens are used, radiographic sharpness decreases, and this trend worsens as faster screens are used (see Figure 63).

Modulation Transfer Function

In brief, modulation transfer function (M.T.F.) refers to the manner in which the phosphors transmit their light to the film. The film, of course, is responsible for receiving the pattern of emitted light intensities and makes a permanent image of them (see Figure 64). Here we see how screen phosphors react to varying intensities of the remnant beam and produce proportionate or representative amounts of light, which in turn will produce proportionate or representative densities on the film. The varying amounts of x-rays striking the phosphors are caused by variations in tissue absorption. M.T.F. is the process of transferring the information of the remnant beam to the emulsion of the x-ray film.

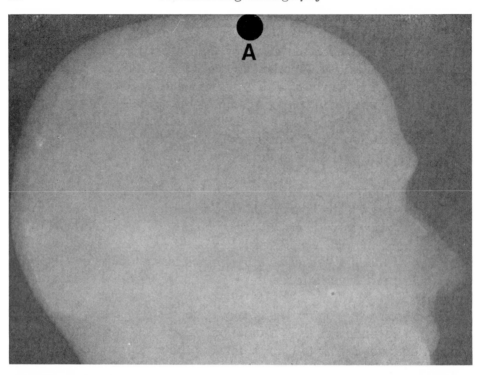

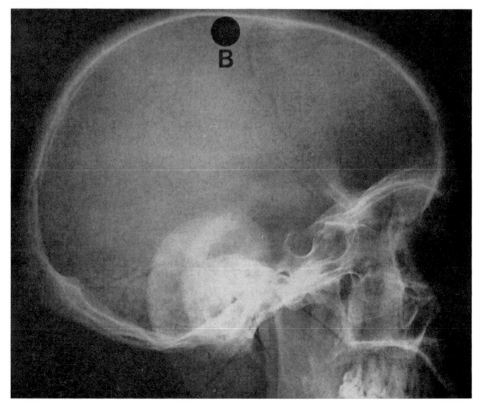

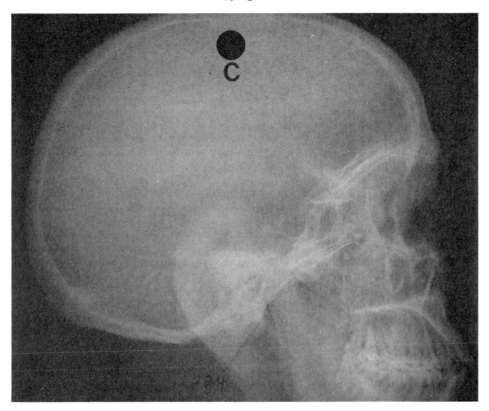

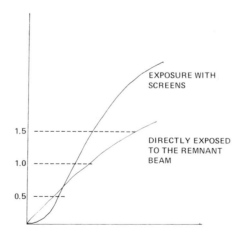

← Figure 61. To show changes in radiographic density, compare *B* using a screen exposure with *A* using a nonscreen exposure. The density in *B* was equalized in *C*, so the difference between these images shows changes in contrast caused by the screen. H & D curves are included for evaluation.

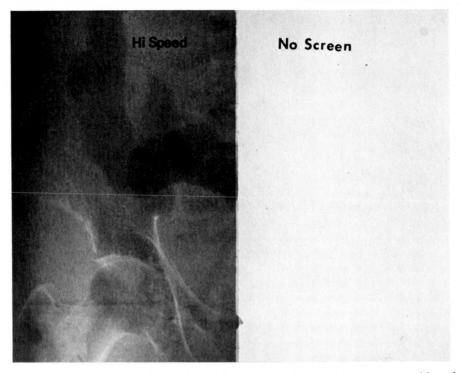

Figure 62. Obtaining quality radiographs without the use of screens would make routine radiography impossible. Compare the radiographic effect of a high speed screen and a nonscreen exposure. A sheet of paper was used to block the screen to one-half of the film.

M.T.F. is the fundamental factor that influences screen unsharpness. In Figure 65, a beam is exposing a film, which responds accordingly and represents the body structures very faithfully. This situation will, of course, produce optimal image sharpness. In other words, there is a one to one transfer of patient information carried by the remnant beam to the film. This, unfortunately, is not the case when intensifying screens are used, because the information transferred to the film is not direct from the patient. There are three factors that affect image transfer: the manner with which the photons emit light, the thickness of the active layer, and the reflective layer.

It has already been discussed how a typical phosphor emits light in all directions, similar to a light bulb. It is obvious what might happen to a sharply defined body structure if a medium that carried the information had a spreading effect as it traveled toward the film. Also, the active layer is made up of phosphors coated to a certain thickness: unsharpness would become worse if *many* crystals carrying the body information had been

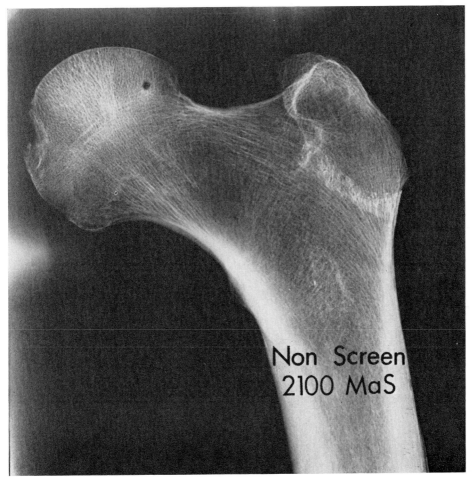

Figure 63A.

Figure 63. Sharpness decreases when changing from nonscreen to screen exposures; further decreases in sharpness result as faster screens are used.

affected by a spreading medium. The factors that influence the degree of the spreading effect are the thickness of the active layer and the efficiency of the reflective layer. Figure 66 illustrates how varying degrees of light spread affect radiographic sharpness. Although the screen's spreading effect is influenced by the thickness of the active layer and the efficiency of the reflective layer, it should be understood that the initial cause of the spreading effect is the inherent pattern of light emission from the crystal itself. A method has been devised with which screens can be tested to determine the degree of spreading ability (M.T.F.) Figure 67 shows two lead blocks precisely cut and separated by a tiny space. Three exposures were made: The nonscreen exposure faithfully duplicated the

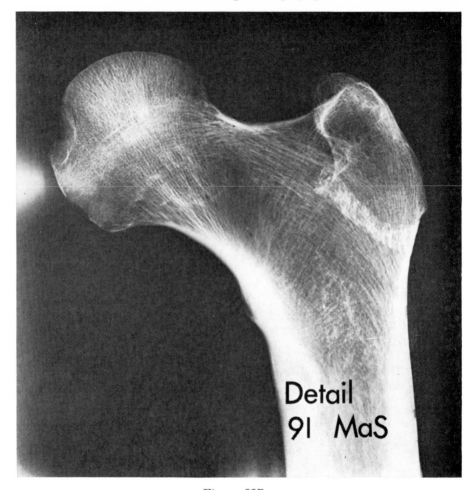

Figure 63B.

sharpness between the block; The slow speed screen gave evidence of a slight spreading function as the film has a wider line of exposure; and fast screens caused increased spreading resulting in the greatest amount of unsharpness.

In summary, modulation transfer function is the process by which the phosphors emit light to the film in a spreading fashion, which cause a loss of structure delineation. As the screen's speed increases, the spreading factor increases and sharpness decreases. It is interesting to note that the size of the crystal has no practical effect on screen sharpness because small phosphors emit light in the same diversion pattern as large ones do. A small crystal must produce the same amount of light as a large crystal to produce equal radiographic density, so a small crystal would eventually have equal spreading if a comparable density is to be maintained.

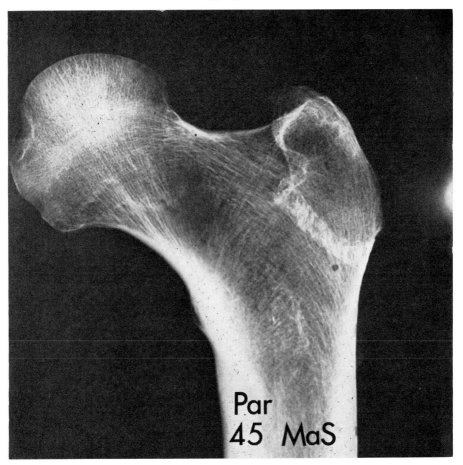

Par
45 MaS

Figure 63C.

Factors Affecting Screen Speed

The prime factors that affect the intensification factor (speed) of screens are the thickness of the active layer, the efficiency of the reflective layer, and the amount of yellow dye* in the active layer. Much discussion has been made regarding the effect changes in KvP have on screen speed; however, the author has found that most conventional phosphors (calcium tungstate) used today are fairly consistent light emitters over the diagnostic KvP range.

The thicker the active layer, the faster the screen will be. The reason for this is that thicker active layers will simply contain more phosphors and thus emit a greater amount of light. In other words, more crystals

---

* Some dyes used to absorb emitted screen light are brown or pink depending on the manufacturer.

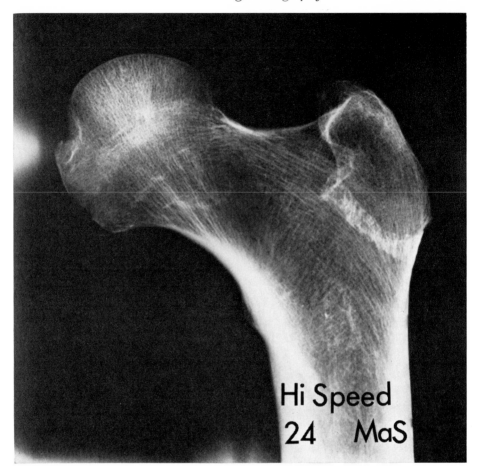

Figure 63D.

will capture or intercept more x-ray photons. This, of course, will make a darker radiograph with the same exposure. A reflective layer has been included in the screen's structure to bounce the escaping light toward the x-ray film. Thus, more screen light reaches the film per a given exposure resulting in a darker image, and, as the efficiency of the reflective layer increases, radiographic density increases. Blue light is absorbed very well by yellow substances. Some screens, usually the slow speed type, appear to be colored. Often this is the main difference between the various speeds of screens. Fast screens are usually white in appearance.

These dyes *artificially* reduce the spreading characteristic of the emitted light resulting in a positive affect on screen and image sharpness. To a lesser extent, atmospheric conditions play a role in affecting screen speed. As air temperature increases, the efficiency of a screen's ability to

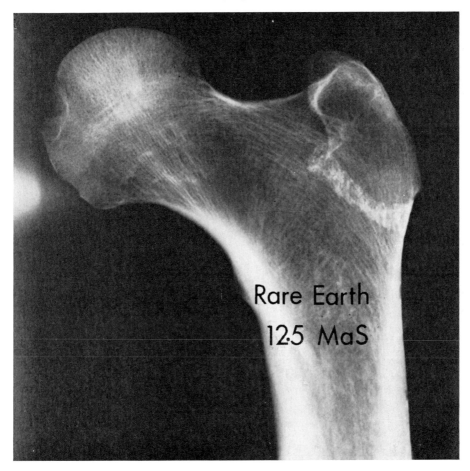

Figure 63E.

produce light decreases; however, film becomes more sensitive to exposure when used in warmer temperatures. The net effect of these opposing conditions between film and screen is that the radiographic density produced by the screen film exposure system remains fairly constant throughout most atmospheric conditions likely to be experienced in the United States.

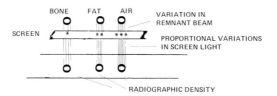

Figure 64. Screens transfer light intensities to the film, which are in turn representative of remnant beam intensities.

MODULATION TRANSFER FUNCTION

(Screen Unsharpness)

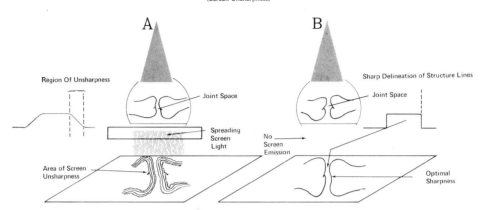

Figure 65. *B* shows that optimal sharpness has been attained because of the one-to-one transference of information carried by the remnant beam to the film. However, *A* shows a dramatic reduction in sharpness because a screen has been inserted. The screen is an intermediary which produces divergent light rays of its own which cause unsharpness.

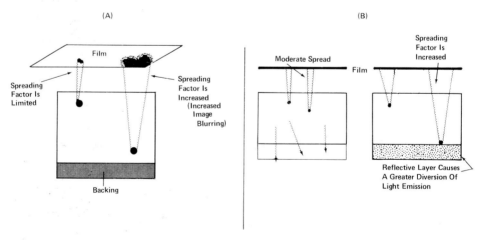

Figure 66. The normal spreading of screen light can be altered by the thickness of the active layer and the efficiency of the reflective layer. As these two factors increase, the spreading factor also increases.

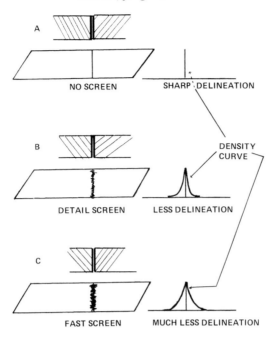

Figure 67. Schematic of modulation transfer. As faster screens are used, the image is more dependent on screen light, and sharpness decreases.

It might be noted, however, that upon freezing a pair of screens overnight and exposing them with film of room temperature, little change in density was noted, compared to the same screen allowed to warm to room temperature and exposed to another film.

Screen Artifacts

There are three fundamental ways in which screens produce artifacts on the radiographic image. One is the obstruction of blue light from the film; under these conditions of obstruction, the film will yield little or no density in that immediate area. Second, screens help to produce static electricity. These charges often expose the film and cause plus $(+)$ density artifacts. Third, poor screen contact is a more subtle artifact, nonetheless equally important as it accounts for a drastic reduction in sharpness.

With regard to the first item, if a foreign object finds its way between the film and screen surfaces and has the ability to absorb the screen's light, a minus density artifact would be caused. Examples of this are noted in Figure 68. Here we see an assortment of paper, hair, and particles of lint placed in the cassette to produce artifacts. Other minus density artifacts caused by light obstruction include stained screens and scratches.

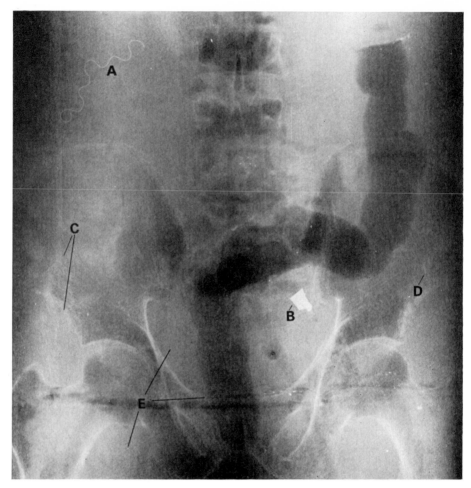

Figure 68. Foreign bodies, artifacts, absorb screen light; the film is not exposed. A—hair; B—paper; C—developer stain; D—scratched screens; E—dirt in cassette.

Screens do lose speed if used too long, but it is not because the phosphors have become less effective. Often, screens lose speed with age because the material used to suspend the phosphor crystal discolors and dries with time to a yellow tint. The blue light is easily absorbed by this discoloration of the suspension material resulting in less blue light getting to the film. There is nothing the technologist can do to correct this except to purchase new screens. Most often, speed is reduced because the abrasion layer is worn away by tiny specks of dirt and foreign material as the film is slid over the screen's surfaces while loading and unloading the cassette. When the abrasion layer is worn away, a layer of dirt forms a barrier to the screen light on route to the film and causes underexposure. From a practical point of view, this would seriously affect quality control because it is possible for the same type of screen to have different speeds if the screens were purchased at different times. The older screens would have more discoloration and artifacts and would yield less radiographic density than the newer ones.

With regard to static, if the screens are not cleaned often enough and were not coated with antistatic solution, friction will result when the film is slid into and out of the cassette. During warm, semihumid atmospheric conditions, static does not usually occur; however, during the winter months, when the air in the department has become dry through heating, friction easily causes static discharges which expose the film as noted in Figure 69. This artifact can be relieved considerably by using a reliable cleaning and antistatic application program. For smaller departments, offices, and clinics, the use of a humidifer could certainly prove beneficial in reducing static problems.

The phosphors located closer to the film surface will produce less light spreading because of their proximity to the film than those located deeper in the active layer. The more distance between the phosphors and the film, the greater the spreading factor will be (as noted in Fig. 70). Because of various problems a cassette might not be able to provide ample compression to assure that the surfaces between the film and screen will be in perfect contact. When this happens, light spreads over a wide area of the film surface causing an obvious decrease in image sharpness. Common causes for this poor contact artifact are: (1) worn felt padding, (2) loose cassette straps, (3) warped or bent cassette frames, (4) cassettes that have developed ridges with use, and (5) expanding and contracting cardboard backing.

A test for poor screen contact involves the use of a wire mesh with approximately one-fourth inch squares, the cassette under suspicion, and a light radiographic exposure: Load a film into the cassette suspected of poor contact, place the wire mesh over the front of the cassette, and make an exposure using approximately 100 Ma, 1/20 second at 50 KvP for high speed screens. When viewing the processed film the white squares of the wire mesh should be sharply defined. If poor screen contact is present, there will be localized patches of unsharpness and slightly increased density over the area. If it is found that the cassette frame is bent or warped, little can be done to improve the problem. If it is simply a matter of worn felt or loose straps, repairs can be made. If the screen itself has ridges, they must be replaced. The day light system by DuPont and the X-Omatic system by Eastman Kodak improve compression substantially. If compression is a problem, it will usually occur in large cassette sizes because it is more difficult to maintain equal compression over this large surface of film area.

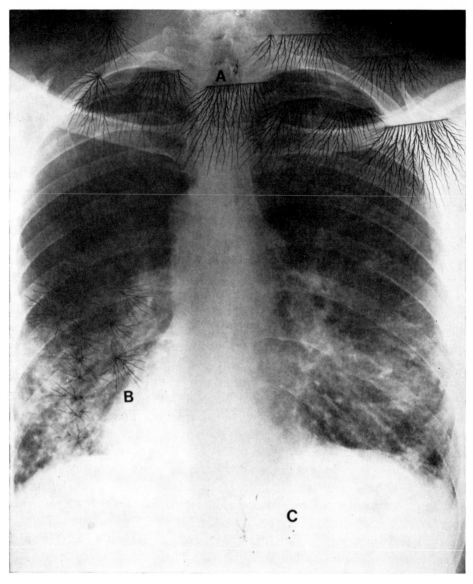

Figure 69. A—crown static; B—"tree" static; C—smudge static. Crown and "tree" static are commonly caused by friction between the film and another surface and are the most common to screens. Smudge static is usually caused by charged dirt and lint particles striking the film.

A less occurring artifact is screen lag. Screen lag is a situation in which the phosphors continue to emit light after transmission of the x-ray exposure (phosphorescence). The phosphors commonly used in making intensifying screens (calcium tungstate) do not phosphoresce. Earlier phosphors had this problem but, fortunately, with the development and

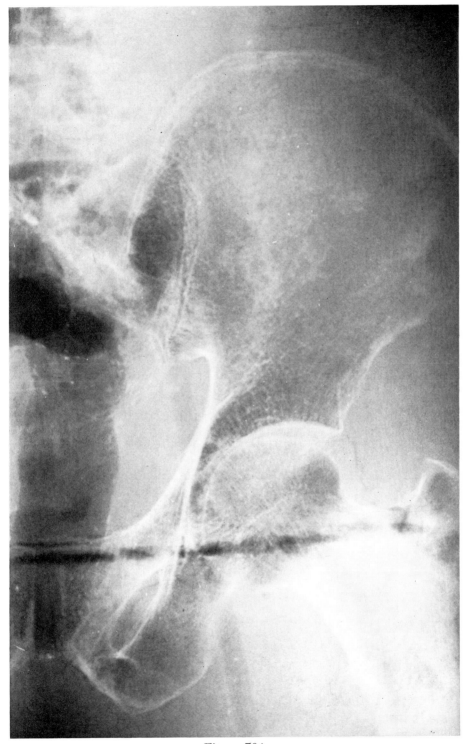

Figure 70A.

Figure 70. Poor screen contact emphasizes the inherent spreading factor of screens, causing additional unsharpness.

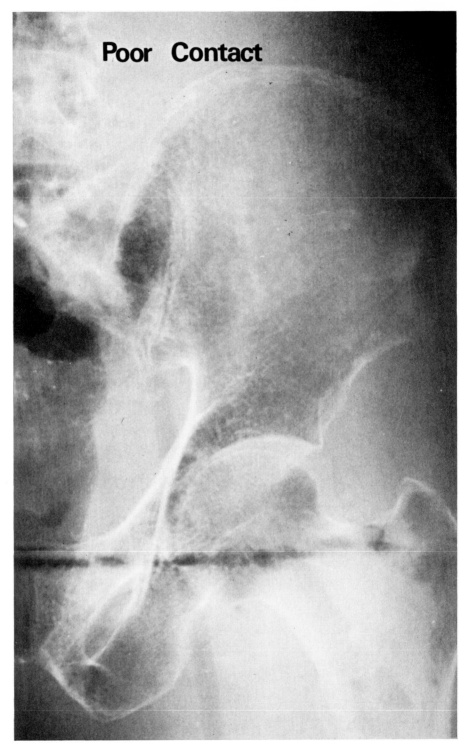

Figure 70B.

SCREEN FILM CONTACT

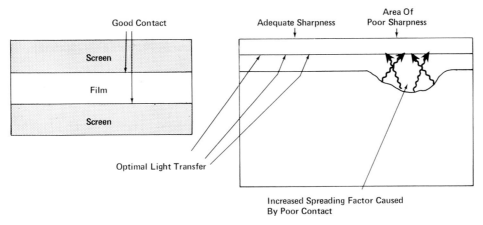

Figure 70C.

advances made with calcium tungstate, screen lag is extremely uncommon in modern radiography.

Quantum Mottle (Noise)

Quantum mottle and screen noise are one and the same. As discussed in physics, x-rays are emitted from an x-ray tube in the form of packettes or individual units of energy called *quantum* (see Fig. 71). In order to get a high quality radiographic image, it is important to have a sufficient amount of quantum to pass through the patient so that enough patient information can be transferred to the film. If not enough quantum (x-rays) are generated during an exposure, an insufficient amount of information will be transferred to the screens and film, and detail will be reduced.

To illustrate this point, Figure 73 shows what happens with quantum mottle. In A a direct exposure is made. A tremendous number of x-rays (quantum) pass through the body picking up large amounts of diagnostic information. This information is directly impressed in the film's emulsion. Because a large number of x-rays were used by the exposure, a representative amount of diagnostic information can be seen on the processed film. In B the situation is somewhat different. Because of the screen's high intensification factor, fewer x-rays are needed to produce equal radiographic density. One can easily see that the amount of useful diagnostic information transmitted to the film via the screen will decrease as the number of x-rays needed to produce a given density decrease. As faster screens are used, still fewer x-ray photons are used to produce the desired density and a greater loss of diagnostic information results. A mottled

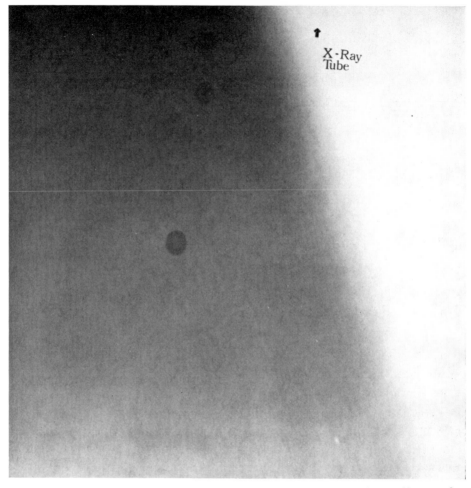

X-Ray
Tube

Figure 71. This exposure was made without a collimator and with the film standing on end under the x-ray tube. One can easily imagine individual quanta exiting the tube and traveling down to expose the film while carrying patient information.

appearance is noted on the film as a result of insufficient numbers of x-ray photons, and is referred to as quantum mottle.

Screen manufacturers were at the point where any further increases in the intensification factor would not be practical because an exposure with still fewer numbers of x-rays could not carry enough information to the screen and film to produce good diagnostic results and the mottled appearance would increase (see Fig. 72). As shown, fewer photons are needed to form a comparable image. These structures could be a part of bone or lung detail in a radiographic image. If superfast screens are used, fewer numbers of x-rays would be needed and the structure would not be seen as well. Quantum mottle appears on the film as faint blotches in the image, especially noticeable when fast screens are used with high KvP exposures.

Rare Earth Screens

It was mentioned earlier that the phosphors' ability to absorb x-ray photons and transfer that energy to visible light is vital to screen radiography. However, as just discussed, when screens become too efficient (fast) quantum mottle occurs and results in a loss of detail. Conventional screens do not absorb all the x-ray photons striking the active layer. Many x-rays are not captured by the phosphors and pass on not converted. Thus much diagnostic information is wasted or unused even though the original film density has been maintained.

Recently, however, new phosphors have been developed as a result of the aerospace program and have become known as rare earth phosphors. This term is slightly misleading as it implies the phosphors are not easily found. Actually, these phosphors are abundant; it is the process under which the phosphors must go in order to be used in intensifying screens that make them less available and thus the term rare earth. There is also a considerable difference in cost between conventional screens and rare earth screens. A conventional pair of calcium tungstate 14 × 17 inch screens lists for approximately 50 percent of the cost if compared to rare earth screens.

The advantage of these screens simply lies in their ability to capture more of the x-rays that have penetrated the body. In fact the capture ratio is approximately double. In other words, conventional fast screens use or capture only 20 percent of the remnant photons, while rare earth screens capture or absorb 40 percent, so rare earth screens can extract twice as much information from the remnant beam than had been previously possible with conventional screens. Quantum mottle is not easily seen even though rare earth screens are twice as fast as conventional high speed screens because more patient information is transferred to the film.

With the increase in capture ratio of these rare earth screens, they can produce twice the amount of light when compared to fast screens, so the exposure can be cut in half—if the original radiographic density is to be maintained. A reduction in exposure in this case would not cause quantum mottle because the screens are absorbing twice as much diagnostic information from the beam.

In summary, rare earth screens allow the technologist to reduce the exposure time by approximately one-half (if compared to fast screens) without any noticeable increase in quantum mottle. This is accomplished with the superior ability of rare earth phosphors to capture or intercept more x-ray photons carrying diagnostic information from the body.

Screen Maintenance

Even under the best of conditions, screens can be expected to last no more than five to six years; thus a good maintenance program should

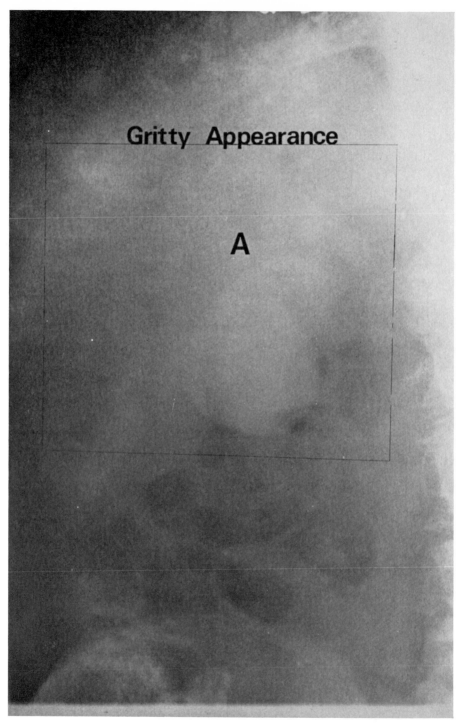

Figure 72. As faster screens are used, fewer primary x-ray photons are necessary to produce sufficient radiographic density. With the decrease in the total number of primary x-ray photons, a proportionate decrease in "patient" information reaches the film.

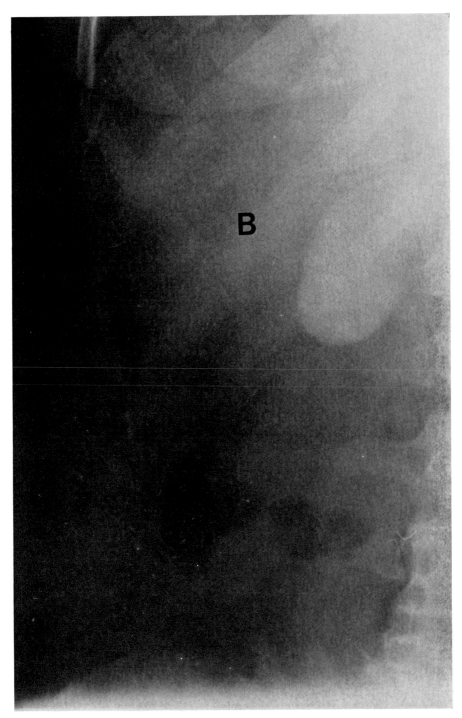

When rare earth screens are used "patient" information reaching the film is not sharply reduced, however, when compared to what occurs with fast screens. The reason for this is that rare earth crystals can capture two times more "patient" information from the remnant beam. The "gritty" appearance in *A* is known as quantum or screen mottle.

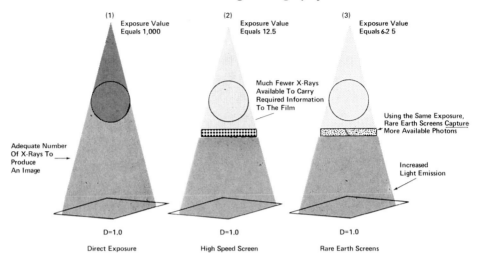

Figure 73. Exposure (1) requires a great many photons because it is a direct exposure; as a result, more "patient" information is carried by the remnant beam to the film. In exposure (2) there is a drastic decrease in the number of photons and less "patient" information is transmitted to the film. In exposure (3), rare earth screens are used. Rare earth screens require approximately 50 percent fewer photons than fast screens but absorb twice as much remnant radiation; thus the same amount of patient information reaches the film.

be enforced. There are many variables in screen usage, and it would be impossible to presume a standard program here. First, the number of screens in the department should be appreciated. If the particular institution has an insufficient supply, they will be used more frequently and consequently require more cleaning and damage will result more readily.

It seems reasonable that screens should be cleaned monthly or bimonthly. A cleaning program helps to prolong the life and prevent the breakdown of the abrasion layer. If screens are not cleaned often enough, lint, dirt, and other hard foreign substances find their way into the screens, and if not removed, will cause scratches as x-ray film is slid in and out of the cassette. Eventually these particles will grind away at the abrasion layer and become embedded into the phosphor layer. Not only has the diagnostic value been reduced substantially, but the screens are costly to replace.

Cleaning instructions are well outlined in the various products designed for the job. It is important, however, not to use too much solution at any one time so that fluid will not seep into the felt padding, and to make sure the screens stand open long enough after cleaning to dry sufficiently (at least twenty minutes).

Nonscreen Versus Screen Film

Film manufacturers can make film more sensitive to certain electromagnetic energy forms; the two major types of film available for radiography purposes are screen and nonscreen film. Screen film is particularly sensitive to blue light. This type can become readily exposed by the emitted light from intensifying screens. Screen-type film can be exposed by the x-ray beam itself, but considerably more exposure must be used to yield the same degree of radiographic density. On the other hand, direct-exposure-type film, also known as nonscreen film, would yield no density if it were exposed with intensifying screens.

The emulsion thickness of screen film should not be great because the blue light from the screens cannot penetrate the silver bromide emulsion very easily. For this reason, screen film is made with emulsion on both sides of the base and is coated more thinly than nonscreen film. If nonscreen film was used in cardboard and screen film was used in cardboard, the nonscreen exposure can be reduced to one-fourth.

New advances in detail with screen radiography in recent years have encouraged more radiologists and technologists to use slow speed screens for high detail work than nonscreen techniques. There is speculation that, in the future, this trend will continue even more, to the extent that nonscreen radiography as we know it will be virtually eliminated.

CHAPTER FIVE

MILLIAMPERAGE

DEFINITION AND FUNCTION

MILLIAMPERAGE IS AN electrical term and not primarily a radiological term. Nevertheless, as you continue through this chapter you will begin to appreciate a vital relationship between the two. For our purposes, milliamperage is the quantity of electrons moving through the x-ray tube during an exposure. A term that is often used in substitution of milliamperage is tube current. The technologist has a great deal of control over the milliamperage. Although Ma indicates the quantity of electrons moving (current), we must be careful to understand that there is no mention of the speed at which the electrons may be moving. If this distinction is noted now, it will help the student to understand the more involved ideas that will be discussed later in the text. In short, the technologist adjusts the milliamperage setting to establish the desired quantity of electrons that will strike the anode of the x-ray tube during the exposure to produce various quantities of primary radiation. There is a relationship between the number of electrons striking the anode and the amount of x-rays that will be produced.

Before any attempt is made to discuss specific details, the following ideas and concepts should be firmly established. We will begin by reviewing a small section of the main x-ray circuit. Figure 74 shows a schematic of the filament circuit. The connection between the control panel and the filament circuit is drastically simplified here, but will serve well in this discussion.

You will note that, at the control panel, a knob is marked Ma selector. Through this control knob the technologist has control over the amount of current that will move in the filament circuit and eventually through the x-ray tube. The panel in Figure 74 also shows that the various Ma values are commonly broken into increments of 50, 100, 200, 300, etc. Modern panels can have Ma values as high as 1,500.

There is a relationship between the position of the milliamperage selector on the control panel and the current that is moving through the filament circuit. In fact, if the technologist moves the milliamperage

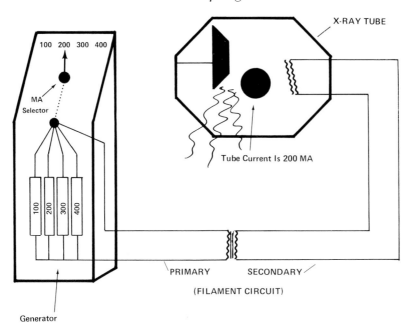

Figure 74. The filament circuit carries current to heat the x-ray tube filament so it will produce proper tube current. The x-ray tube uses the space charge provided by the filament circuit and the high voltage supplied by the high tension circuit to produce x-rays. As the filament temperature increases, more electrons are available to be used as tube current when the technologist presses the exposure switch.

control knob from the 200 Ma station to the 400 Ma station, the amount of current that will move through the filament circuit rises sufficiently to increase the radiographic density by approximately two times (see Fig. 78).

The X-Ray Tube Filament

In order to make practical radiographic use of the filament current it must be channeled by the filament circuit to something that will use these electrons for radiographic purposes. The device used is, of course, the x-ray tube. The x-ray tube will change the energy bound electrons of the filament circuit into x-ray energy (see Fig. 75).

In Figure 76, you will note that the x-ray tube has two major electrodes known as the cathode (which has a negative charge) and the anode (which has a positive charge). Another name given to the cathode is the filament, which resembles the filament of an ordinary light bulb. You will also note that the filament is actually part of the filament circuit while the anode is a part of the high tension circuit. It might be helpful to think of the x-ray tube as a bridge between two different circuits. If the

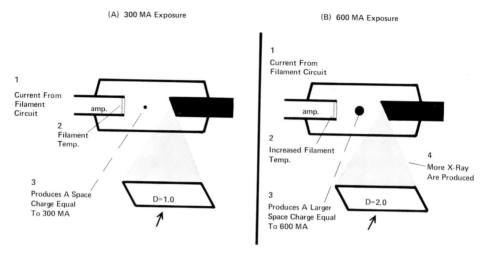

Figure 75.

technologist turns up the Ma selector at the control panel, more current will pass through the filament circuit, and this will increase the temperature of the filament in the x-ray tube. If we increase the filament temperature, the filament's atoms will become so active that it will not be able to contain all its electrons, and they will begin to "boil off" and form a small space charge just beyond the filament. This boiling-off process is often referred to as incandescence and is controlled by the temperature of the filament (see Fig. 75).

When the boiling process begins at the heated filament, the freed electrons have a tendency to remain in a relatively tight ball or cloud just beyond the cathode. The size of the cloud has an important relation-

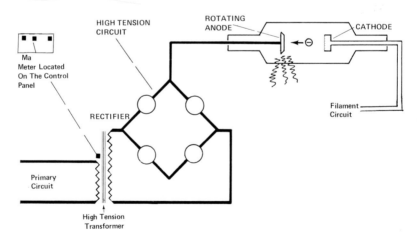

Figure 76.

ship with the temperature of the filament. As the filament temperature is increased, the size of the space charge increases, and when a larger cloud of electrons moves during the exposure, the tube current increases accordingly.

The conversion of electric energy into x-ray energy involves three factors: (1) a space charge must be generated; (2) the electron cloud must be put into motion; (3) once in motion the cloud of electrons must be abruptly stopped. Figure 76 shows that the filament (cathode) is part of the filament circuit and the anode is part of the high tension circuit. These two electrodes function as two coordinated yet separate entities in producing the desired effect of converting electrical kinetic energy into x-ray energy.

As the cloud of electrons is formed, it must be given a great deal of kinetic energy. The anode is thus given a strong positive charge by the high tension circuit. When the technologist presses the exposure button, the secondary circuit closes and the cloud of electrons (space charge) is driven toward the anode at a very high rate of speed. The *Ma meter* at the control panel then registers the quantity of current moving through the x-ray tube. This sequence of events is possible because opposite electrical charges attract each other. The final phase in the production of x-rays involves the stopping or deceleration of the electron cloud with its great amount of kinetic energy. Figure 77 shows the shape of the rotating anode. Because the anode material has a very high atomic number, it is very effectively able to stop the electrons momentarily. The kinetic energy does not simply disappear at this point but rather changes into two other energy forms: heat energy and x-ray energy (the law of conservation of energy). The number of electrons in the space charge will determine to a great extent the number of conversions that occur and the number of x-rays that will emerge as a result.

As Ma selection increases, filament current increases, filament temperature increases, space charge increases, Ma increases, and x-ray and heat production increase.

It can be seen that the technologist can exert direct control over the number of x-rays that will ultimately be produced. It should be kept in mind also that changes in Ma only alter the numbers (quantity) of primary x-rays and not the penetrating ability (see Fig. 78).

It was mentioned that milliamperage is the number of electrons moving in unison through the tube. Often students have the impression that milliamperage indicates a large quantity of electrons when actually it does not. "Milli" means one-thousandth of, so when a 500 Ma station is selected, only ½ amps are used. One must be careful not to underestimate, how-

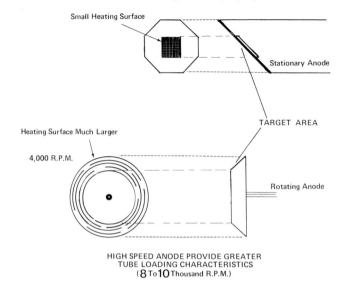

Figure 77. The anode of the x-ray tube contains a target or focal spot which is the site of actual electron bombardment and kinetic energy transformation into primary x-ray photons.

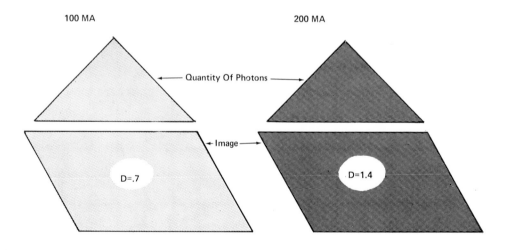

Figure 78. As more photons are produced, radiographic density increases. Radiographs do not always respond as shown here because of other variables such as film speed, specific processing conditions, and whether or not screens are used. ⋏ number of x-rays = ⋏ ionization = ⋏ growth of sensitivity specks = ⋏ density.

ever, the heat and the number of photons that can be generated at the anode during such an exposure.

Ma, Heat, Focal Spot Size, and Radiographic Sharpness

High milliamperage exposures pose serious limitations on the life of x-ray tubes because of the heat generated at the anode during the exposure. The entire anode is not directly subjected to this intense heat, however. A very small area, known as the focal spot, is the primary *target* of the electron cloud. Most diagnostic x-ray tubes range in focal spot sizes from 0.5 mm to 2 mm. The focal spot represents a conflicting problem, because a small sized focal spot (0.5 mm) produces greater sharpness than does a larger focal spot size. However, the intense heat caused by the electrons striking a small area of the anode can be very damaging. Tube life becomes an important consideration in radiography on the basis of cost. The subject of focal spot size and detail will be further evaluated in Chapter 6. It was mentioned here to point out the fact that the milliamperage used for an exposure has an effect on tube life. The statement below summarizes this concept:

As Ma increases, larger tube currents are generated; larger focal size should be used and sharpness of detail decreases.

From a theoretical point of view, it would be incorrect to say that increasing milliamperage itself causes poor sharpness. It would be quite possible to have *optimal* sharpness with a 1,000 Ma exposure, providing it was possible to use a small focal size. Each new x-ray tube delivered to an installation has a graph that gives the technologist sufficient information regarding safe exposure settings so that tube damage can be avoided. These graphs are very easy to use, but the technologist must be sure that he is using the correct graph for the tube. This can be determined by matching phasing, rectification, and the focal spot size (see Fig. 79).

Reciprocity Law

Considering the possibilities of damaging an x-ray tube because of excessive anode heat, one might question the value of using high milliamperage exposures at all. From the technologist's point of view, the primary significance of using high exposures is that they allow equally short times to be used. If an exposure is made while the subject is in motion, there exists the possibility of a blurred image. In the case of pediatric examinations, it is especially important to use the shortest exposure time possible to reduce the chances of blurring from patient motion. The relationship between exposure time and milliamperage is very nicely bal-

SINGLE RADIOGRAPHIC EXPOSURE RATINGS

SINGLE PHASE – FULL WAVE RECTIFICATION
STANDARD SPEED (60 Hertz)

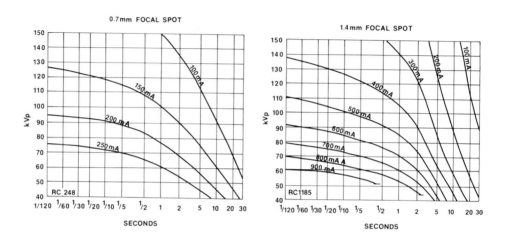

HIGH SPEED (180 Hertz)

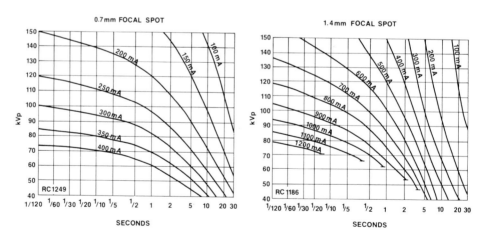

Figure 79: *Courtesy of* Picker X-Ray Corporation.

anced in the phenomenon described by the *Reciprocity Law*. This law refers to a compatibility between the accumulation of radiation on the film caused by beam intensity and exposure time. This relationship is valid, so that some manufacturers of x-ray equipment combine exposure time and Ma factors into one unit known as milliamperage-second (MaS).

MaS is simply the product of the Ma and time value used for a given purpose. Let us examine a common exposure made using 200 Ma at 1 second at 70 KvP. These settings of time and Ma will produce the same radiographic density as 200 MaS at 70 KvP.

$$200 \text{ Ma} \times 1 \text{ sec} = 200 \text{ MaS}$$

From a practical point of view, many technologists find it more convenient to think in terms of MaS when setting techniques than by calculating individual units of time and Ma. The reciprocity between time and Ma can sometimes be better understood if we consider that 200 MaS can be obtained by a wide variety of combinations as noted below (also see Table I):

$$200 \text{ Ma} \times 1 \text{ sec} = 200 \text{ MaS}$$
$$400 \text{ Ma} \times \tfrac{1}{2} \text{ sec} = 200 \text{ MaS}$$
$$800 \text{ Ma} \times \tfrac{1}{4} \text{ sec} = 200 \text{ MaS}$$
$$100 \text{ Ma} \times 2 \text{ sec} = 200 \text{ MaS}$$

Each of the above exposure settings will produce the same accumulation of x-rays striking the film resulting in equal density. Reciprocity between time and Ma exist when direct exposure films are used. There is a slight breakdown in reciprocity with intensifying screens. This reciprocity failure occurs with very short or very long exposure times: less than 1/120 of a second or greater than 5 seconds. It should be noted that the slight degree of reciprocity failure is usually not serious enough to cause practical technical problems.

MILLIAMPERAGE CALIBRATION

The technologist often has to make adjustments from what the technique charts indicate. For example, suppose an abdomen examination is to be done, and the patient requires 80 KvP, 100 Ma, at ½ second; because of the patient's inability to suspend respiration, it is necessary to decrease the exposure time but maintain overall radiographic density. Recalling the reciprocity law one may then use 400 Ma at ⅛ of a second. This would accomplish the desired result, providing the x-ray equipment is properly calibrated to produce 400 Ma accurately. In many generators, however, this is not the case. Occasionally the x-ray output of a specific Ma is out of calibration so that when 400 Ma is selected, the actual output may be 350 or sometimes even less. If a technologist is working with an uncalibrated generator, equal densities will not result at the same MaS values and the technologist will end up making repeat exposures. Figure 80 shows radiographs exposed with the same generator before and after proper adjustments were made in Ma calibrations. Since the tube

TABLE I

MaS CALCULATIONS

Pulses	Time	50	100	200	300	400	500	600	700	800	900	1000	1100	1200	1300	1400	1500
1	1/120::	0.4	0.8	1.6	2.5	3	4	5	5	6	7	8	9	10	10	11	12
2	1/60::	0.8	1.6	3.2	5.0	6	8	10	11	13	15	16	18	20	21	23	25
3	1/40::	1.2	2.5	5.0	7.5	10	12	15	17	20	22	25	27	30	32	35	37
4	1/30::	1.6	3.3	6.6	10	13	16	20	23	26	29	33	36	39	43	46	49
5	1/24::	2	4	8	12	16	20	25	29	33	37	41	45	50	54	58	62
6	1/20::	2.5	5	10	15	20	25	30	35	40	45	50	55	60	65	70	75
8	1/15::	3.3	6.6	13	20	26	33	40	46	53	60	66	73	80	86	93	100
10	1/12::	4.1	8.3	16	25	33	41	50	58	66	75	83	91	100	108	116	125
12	1/10::	5	10	20	30	40	50	60	70	80	90	100	110	120	130	140	150
15	1/8::	6.2	12.5	25	37	50	62	75	87	100	112	125	137	150	162	175	187
18	3/20::	7.5	15	30	45	60	75	90	105	120	135	150	165	180	195	210	225
20	1/6::	8	16	33	50	66	83	100	116	133	150	166	183	200	216	233	250
24	2/10::	10	20	40	60	80	100	120	140	160	180	200	220	240	260	280	300
30	1/4::	12.5	25	50	75	100	125	150	175	200	225	250	275	300	325	350	375
	3/10::	15	30	60	90	120	150	180	210	240	270	300	330	360	390	420	450
	7/20::	17	35	70	105	140	175	210	245	280	315	350	385	420	455	490	525
	4/10::	20	40	80	120	160	200	240	280	320	360	400	440	480	520	560	600
	9/20::	22	45	90	135	180	225	270	315	360	405	450	495	540	585	630	675
	1/2::	25	50	100	150	200	250	300	350	400	450	500	550	600	650	700	750
	11/20::	27	55	110	165	220	275	330	385	440	495	550	605	660	715	770	825
	6/10::	30	60	120	180	240	300	360	420	480	540	600	660	720	780	840	900
	13/20::	32	65	130	195	260	325	390	455	520	585	650	715	780	845	910	975
	7/10::	35	70	140	210	280	350	420	490	560	630	700	770	840	910	980	1050
	6/8::	37	75	150	225	300	375	450	525	600	675	750	825	900	975	1050	1125
	8/10::	40	80	160	240	320	400	480	560	640	720	800	880	960	1040	1120	1200
	9/10::	45	90	180	270	360	450	540	630	720	810	900	990	1080	1170	1260	1350
	1SEC::	50	100	200	300	400	500	600	700	800	900	1000	1100	1200	1300	1400	1500
	1 1/4::	62	125	250	375	500	625	750	875	1000	1125	1250	1375	1500	1625	1750	1875
	1 1/2::	75	150	300	450	600	750	900	1050	1200	1350	1500	1650	1800	1950	2100	2250

Milliamperage

current (Ma) is so vital to the x-ray exposure, the technologist should watch the Ma meter during the exposure. If the Ma selector is placed at 300 Ma for a given exposure, the Ma meter should read 300 during the exposure and the MaS meter for very short exposures. For various reasons, problems can arise throughout the x-ray circuits that would cause the meter to read slightly higher or lower. If this variation in Ma reading is great, the x-ray generator should be recalibrated by a competent service person. In retrospect, this is frequently the reason why technique charts do not always work: the chart might call for 400 Ma, but the generator was actually producing 275 which will yield an underexposed image.

If the Ma meter makes no reading at all, there simply is no tube current and no x-ray photons are produced. This can happen as a result of the Kv or Ma selectors not being properly seated. To remedy this, the technologist should simply turn the selectors a few stops over and then back again to the original setting. The milliamperage meter can also indicate what is known as a gassy tube. In this condition, the x-ray tube for various reasons has lost its vacuum to air and during the exposure not only the desired cloud of electrons move toward the anode but a high amount of *electrons* from the air as well. This produces a tremendous volume of tube current and the Ma meter will "spike" as it monitors the additional current moving through the tube. When this occurs the x-ray unit should be turned off immediately and a supervisor notified.

PATIENT DOSE AND MILLIAMPERAGE

Although the subject of radiation safety is not within the direct scope of this text, some mention should be made that milliamperage does affect patient dose. Very simply stated, when all other things are held constant, the more numbers of individual x-ray photons (primary radiation) used during an exposure, the greater dose the patient receives. An exposure of 200 Ma for one second at 70 KvP will produce two times the radiation dose to the patient than 100 Ma used for one second at 70 KvP.

The term *exposure rate* is often used in a radiological sense to indicate the intensity or concentration of a given x-ray beam. Exposure rate is often expressed in the form of m/r. Under these conditions one could expect to see that twice the number of photons would be produced in the x-ray beam if the exposure was changed from 100 Ma to 200 Ma. The exposure rate would *not* be affected, however, if the *exposure time* were changed from one to two seconds because the intensity or concentration of photons per a given time around the measuring device would not have changed, even though the total accumulative exposure was doubled.

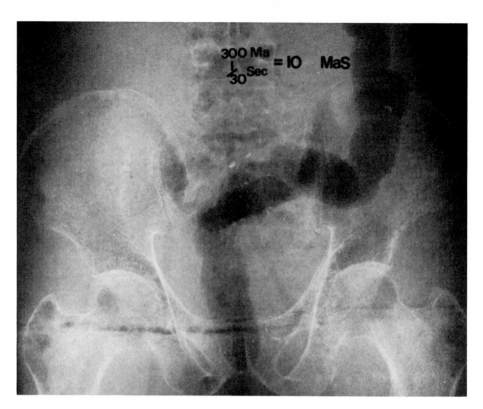

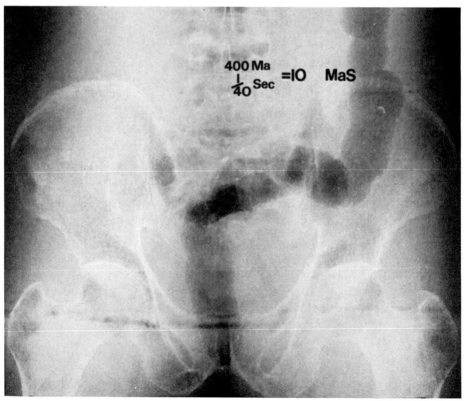

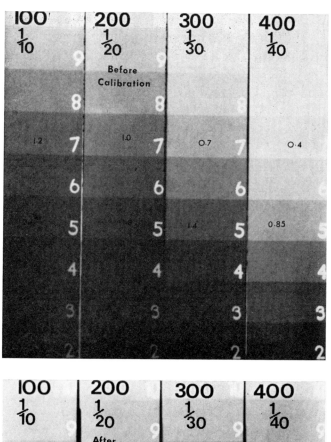

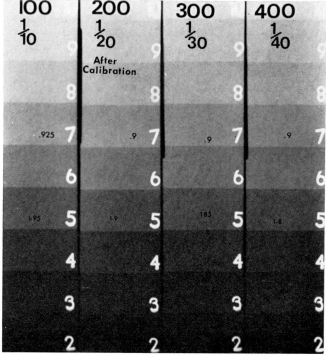

← Figure 80. Both pelvic examinations were exposed with different time and Ma values; however the MaS is equal so radiographic density should be very similar. Accompanying gray scales were made using the same MaS (10) but with different Ma stations. Note the variations on the before and after radiographs.

THE RADIOGRAPHIC EFFECT

Density and Milliamperage

In the previous pages we have discussed how the milliamperage selector is used to control the size of the space charge and how the tube
current relates to the number of x-rays produced during exposure. Although this background is essential for the technologist to successfully
adjust his exposure factors, he must also be able to predict how these
electrical changes in the x-ray circuit will manifest changes in a radiographic image (see Fig. 81). The effect milliamperage has on the radio-

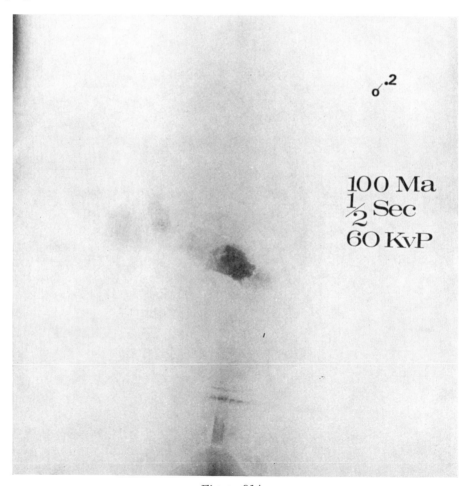

Figure 81A.

Figure 81. As the technologist selects higher Ma stations at the control panel, more
filament heat is created in the x-ray tube and, as a result, a larger space charge is produced. This chain of events causes nearly proportional increases in film density, depending on processing and film type and whether screens are used. This series of
radiographs is made with increasing Ma values.

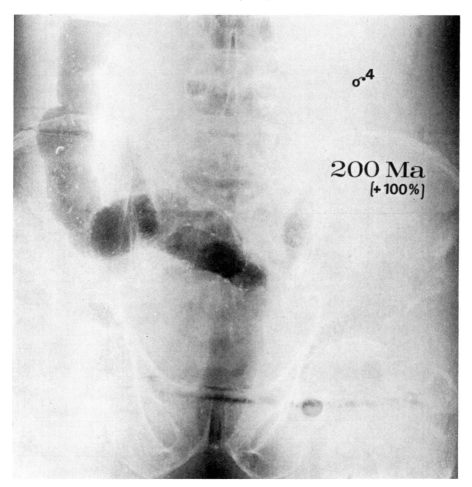

Figure 81B.

graphic image is primarily that of density. As the technologist uses higher Ma settings at the control panel, proportionately more x-rays are produced, resulting in a greater accumulation of x-rays on the film's emulsion. Since radiographic density can be controlled by the amount of x-rays that have exposed the silver bromide crystals, if twice the number of crystals were ionized during an exposure, radiographic density would be doubled.

Contrast and Milliamperage

Within practical terms, milliamperage has no direct effect on radiographic contrast. The reason for this is that, under normal conditions, radiographic contrast is a measure of how evenly or unevenly the various body parts have been penetrated and the rate of scatter that was produced by the patient during the exposure. Because milliamperage has no

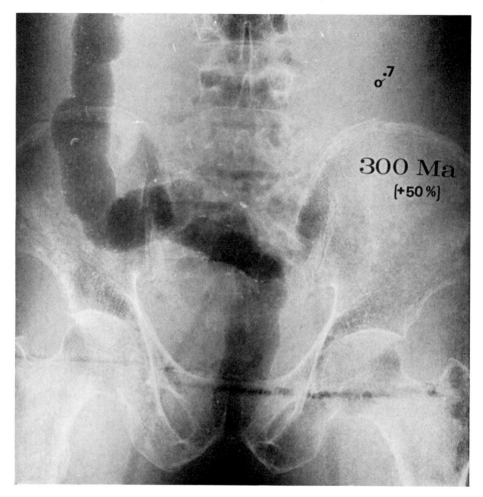

Figure 81C.

influence on these aspects of the x-ray beam, contrast is virtually un-
affected by changing the Ma or the MaS. Figure 81 shows common Ma
exposure values and the resulting effect on density—as the technologist
increased the Ma, more radiation was produced and more silver bromide
crystals were ionized: As a result, the image increased in density. As
increased density occurs, radiographic contrast does not change substantially because the relationship *between* the densities remains fairly constant. As you review these radiographs, keep in mind that there is no
specific agreement, except for extreme cases, as to what level of radiographic density will produce optimal visibility of detail. In general, the
degree of radiographic density desired mostly depends on personal pref-
erence.

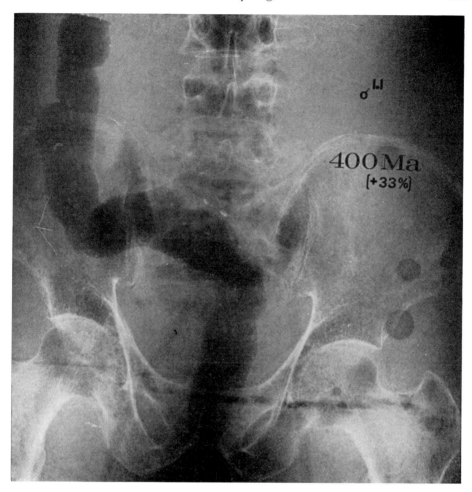

Figure 81D.

EXPOSURE TIME

The function of exposure time is to provide a duration in which the x-ray beam is allowed to irradiate the patient and the film. In general, radiography requires the shortest exposure time possible. The primary reason for this is to reduce the chance of patient motion which results in decreased sharpness. Exposure times commonly range from $\frac{1}{120}$ sec to $1\frac{1}{2}$ sec depending on the examination. Exposure time can have a great effect on the life of the x-ray tube. Extremely short times or very long exposures can cause serious tube damage and thus must be taken into account when establishing technique charts and when calculating single exposures. The technologist should always have a tube rating chart at his disposal so that a given technique can be easily checked if it is suspected of being in the range of the tube limit.

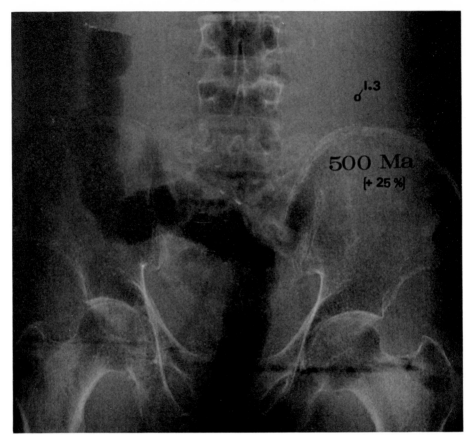

Figure 81E.

Very short times in combination with very intense exposures will cause tube damage as well. The reason for this can be understood if we consider how anode heat is generated. Each pulse of tube current that spurts from the cathode generates a tremendous amount of anode heat which must be dissipated very quickly. The heat is dissipated by the spinning anode and is carried by conduction to other parts of the tube's component parts as seen in Figure 82. If the total exposure necessary for the required image is spaced over one second for example, the total amount of heat generated by each burst of tube current can be properly spread over the entire surface of the spinning anode. If, however, an exposure time of $\frac{1}{40}$ sec was used, the intensity of the tube current must be increased approximately forty times to produce the same total amount of radiation for an equal exposure. This increased intensity of tube current causes a tremendous increase of anode heat which in a long run will decrease life expectancy of the tube or even cause serious damage immediately, depending on the actual exposure factors used and the capacity of the tube. With the ⅟₄₀ sec exposure, the generated heat is not spread as uniformly over the spinning anode. If very short times are routinely used in combination with very intense exposure, uneven anode heat will result which, in turn, will cause uneven expansion of the anode. This condition if continued will eventually produce small cracks on the anode and eventually bring about the demise of the entire tube. It would be very difficult to state categorical rules regarding exposure factors and tube life because of the large number of variables in the type of x-ray tubes.

ANODE HEAT CONDUCTION

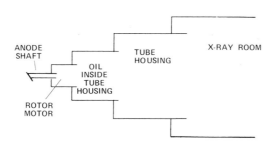

Figure 82. Without a method of anode heat conduction, the x-ray tube would become damaged after only a few exposures. In addition to what is shown, tubes can be purchased that have special oil or water circulating devices.

Some exceptions in the policy of using the short exposures to reduce motion: ribs, lateral thoracic spines, and sternum radiographs make long exposure times very beneficial. A long exposure time will permit enough motion of the surrounding body parts so that they blur, while the body part being studied remains still and more visible.

Exposure Time and the X-ray Beam

Exposure time has no influence on the composition or the characteristics of the x-ray beam. It does not influence the beam's intensity or penetrating power. It does have an obvious effect on radiographic density. As longer exposures are used (assuming all other factors are constant) the accumulation of radiation on the film increases. If exposure time is excessively long, more and more silver bromide crystals will acquire a latent image (become ionized), and radiographic density becomes excessive. Thus, exposure time has a strong influence on visibility of detail because of its effect on radiographic density. It also has some influence on sharpness of detail because of its effect on patient motion. The relationship between exposure time and radiographic density is nearly direct (as will be discussed in Chapter Eleven); however, a number of variables do influence this relationship so that once again a categorical statement regarding the exact effect exposure time has on density cannot be correctly made.

Exposure Time and Scatter Radiation

There is often a misunderstanding regarding the role time has in producing secondary scattered radiation. Scatter radiation (S/S) is somewhat proportional to changes in time and Ma. If a technique of 70 KvP, 100 Ma, at ½ sec is chosen, and the part to be radiographed is an abdomen, the primary to secondary ratio might be 1:7. This ratio will play an important role in the resulting radiographic contrast. If the exposure time is increased to 1 sec, roughly twice the total number of x-rays will pass through the body, causing an increase in radiographic density. However, since the kilovoltage was constant, the type of interactions produced (which is what determines the primary to secondary ratio) would be nearly the same although the numbers would be different, perhaps 2:14.

Automatic Timing Devices

An alternate method of accurately timing the x-ray exposure is commonly called phototiming or automatic timing. It involves the use of a device generally referred to as a photo pickup. It is composed of a small intensifying screen which is positioned in front of a small photoelectric cell. The photoelectric cell is capable of producing a small electric current after it has received a certain amount of light from the intensifying screen. The photoelectric cell is connected to the x-ray circuit in such a way that when it is stimulated by the fluorescent light to a predetermined limit, it will generate enough current to "trip" the exposure switch in the x-ray circuit thus terminating the x-ray exposure. There are many different designs and variations in manufacturing phototiming equipment. A discussion of their individual advantages and disadvantages is not as important as understanding the basic concept and how it relates to the radiographic image.

When using such a device, the technologist need only set the desired KvP (penetration and subject contrast) and Ma. The sensitivity of the photoelectric cell is usually set during the installation and except for minor adjustments left alone. It is the sensitivity of the photoelectric cell to the fluorescent light that determines radiographic density. When the photons strike the tiny fluorescent screen, the screen will give off light. As more photons reach the screen, its light output increases. This continues until it produces enough light to energize the photo cell, which then produces a small current and trips the remote exposure switch.

Automatic timing might at first appear to be a technologist's dream;

however, all the good features are balanced by a few important limitations. One of these is that phototiming often has difficulty in producing consistent radiographs when radiographing patients with a variety of diseases, i.e. excessive water accumulations. If the pickup (the fluorescent screen and photoelectric cell) happens to lie over a tumor for example, very little radiation will reach the screen, and the photocell will not become excited and produce current to signal the exposure switch. With this situation, the exposure will continue endlessly while the other areas of the body are being overexposed. The result of this would be that the film containing other body parts would have been "burned out".

A second limitation to phototiming involves positioning of the body part. With phototiming, the technologist has little positioning latitude. If the pickup is not positioned directly under the body part of interest, the probability is high that the resulting radiograph will be either too light or too dark. If the technologist will remember that the pickup is working "blind" and that it only "reads" the amount of radiation coming from the body part positioned immediately overhead and will control the entire exposure accordingly, it will be easier to understand the relationship between the equipment, positioning of the body part, and resulting radiographic density.

Reaction time of the photoelectric cell and its signal to the exposure switch is another important limitation with phototiming equipment. Reaction time is the total amount of time it takes for the fluorescent screen to emit light, plus the time it takes for the photoelectric cell to send its signal to the x-ray exposure switch, plus the time it takes the exposure switch to finally terminate the exposure. In many modern phototimed systems, regardless of the claims from manufacturers, one should not expect *consistent* automatic exposure control for times less than $\frac{1}{60}$ sec. If a chest examination is to be done on a moderate weight or thin patient using high KvP values of perhaps 140, and the Ma is set at perhaps 300, the exposure time should normally be about $\frac{1}{60}$ second depending on processing, speed of the film, and speed of the screens. However, if a phototiming device is used that has a reaction time of $\frac{1}{30}$ sec, the light from the screen may stimulate the photocell quickly enough, but the other components cannot respond to terminate the exposure before $\frac{1}{30}$ sec has passed. This would, of course, produce approximately twice the radiographic density that is needed. The only adjustment that can be made to compensate for these conditions is to reduce the Ma and/or the KvP. Figure 83 shows the major component parts as they might be arranged in a typical phototiming system. Only the specific body part being monitored for density by the phototimer is located immediately over the phototimer pickup (see Fig. 84).

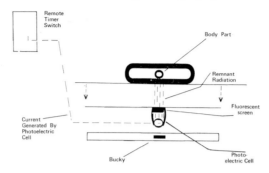

Figure 83.

One last factor is that the manual time selector will automatically override the phototimer device if it is set by error or intentionally to a lesser time value than might be needed by the phototimer. For example, an abdomen exposure is to be done using the phototimer and is automatically terminated at $\frac{4}{10}$ of a second; if the manual timer is set for $\frac{2}{10}$ of a second, it will conclude the exposure at $\frac{2}{10}$ sec. Thus, one must be careful to keep the manual timer selector at a point where it will not conflict with the automatic timing device. It is good practice, however, to keep the manual timer set close to what the automatic exposure will be in case the automatic system fails and a backup timer is needed to prevent a x-ray tube overload.

Despite the limitations pointed out above, automatic timing offers some important advantages. Considering these limitations, the only one

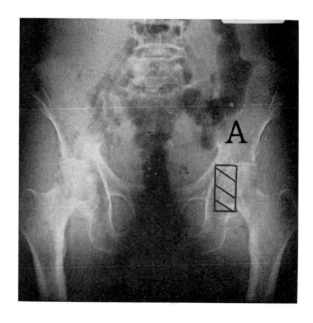

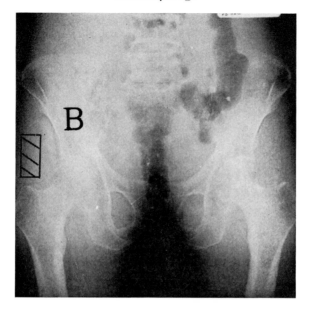

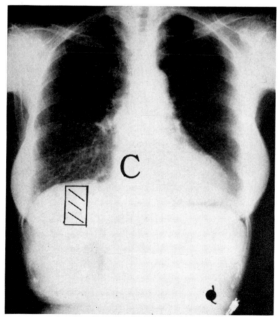

← Figure 84. If the body part is not correctly positioned over the photocell, improper radiographic density will result. In *A*, correct placement produced the desired results. In *B*, acceptable soft tissue density was produced, but the hip is too light because the photocell received enough radiation to terminate the exposure. In *C*, the rib study is too dark because the cell never received enough radiation to excite it and terminate the exposure.

that is beyond the technologist's control are those involving pathology. The technologist can soon master the problem of positioning with a reasonable amount of interest and ability. The major advantage with automatic timing devices is that they provide consistent radiographic densities from one patient to another and, as a result, over-all quality control is considerably more predictable. Because the KvP is held constant for each phototimed exposure, radiographic contrast is also relatively consistent. Along with this, one can assume a lower repeat rate as well, so patient traffic through a busy department can be managed more effectively. This will, in the long run result in a notable improvement in overall efficiency. In short, the phototiming device if properly used and calibrated cannot only improve overall departmental radiographic quality but increase efficiency as well.

CHAPTER SIX

FOCAL FILM DISTANCE

Introduction

THERE REMAINS ONE PRIME factor that has a profound effect on the radiographic image and does so in a much different way. In fact, focal film distance can complicate an exposure to such an extent it is seldom used as a variable when formulating x-ray techniques. In viewing this subject, it might be useful to once again consider a separation or independence between what has been termed the projected beam and the technical beam. If these concepts can be appreciated as two separate entities, and if it is kept in mind that the conditions affecting the projected (or geometric) beam *and* the technical beam must be optimal before a high radiographic image is realized, the study of radiography in general becomes more manageable. The technical beam consists of variation of intensity and quantity of remnant photons.

When the sun's rays shine through the atmosphere they pass many objects. The ability of the rays to pass through clouds of various thickness is primarily what can be considered its technical aspects (quantity and quality). Principally, these involve the frequency or energy of the sun's rays which are caused by the tremendous heat produced from the sun's burning gasses. The energy of the sun's light rays could be related to KvP, and the *amount* of gasses available for burning can be loosely related to the milliamperage if we were to use radiologic terms. As the sun's rays move toward the earth they carry bits of information about the contents of the atmosphere. On a cloudy day, for example, the bright sun is not seen because clouds have absorbed its light and there is some degree of darkness. If, on the other hand, the sun is shining brightly and there are only a few clouds scattered throughout the sky, we will observe shadows, which tell us something is above which the sun's rays are having difficulty penetrating. By observing these shadows, we may be able to tell something about the makeup of the clouds in terms of shape and thickness or density.

THE GEOMETRIC BEAM (OR PROJECTED BEAM)

The common sundial can help explain the projected or geometric beam. The projected beam automatically changes when there is a change in the direction or pattern of the rays emitted by the x-ray tube. Figure 85 shows a sundial and its shadow at various points as the geometry of the sun's rays change throughout the day. The shape and the direction of the shadow produced by the sundial change as the angle of the sun's rays alter in position. Imagine for a moment what might happen to the

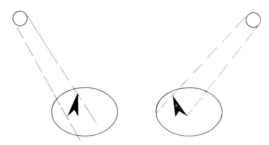

Figure 85. As the sun projects its rays toward the sundial, a geometric pattern (shadow) is projected onto its base. In radiography, similar geometric patterns are responsible for transmitting the various sharply defined structures seen in the radiograph.

radiographic image if the technologist is using the correct technical factors (MaS and KvP) but has incorrectly positioned the angle of the x-ray beam during an examination of a joint space. On reviewing Figure 86, it is easy to see that the position of the tube in A has *closed* the joint space, decreasing the diagnostic value of the examination. Thus, the projected beam affects the shape and the location of the structures seen on radiographs and can produce aberrations (distortions) of the actual body part. In general, such distortions or aberrations are not wanted because they make it very difficult for the radiologist to make a correct interpretation or assessment of the structures under examination.

FOCAL FILM DISTANCE AND THE INVERSE SQUARE LAW

As focal film distance (F.F.D.) increases, radiographic density decreases. The reason for this can be seen in Figure 87. Density readings change as the x-ray tube is moved further from the film. As a prime factor in radiography, focal film distance affects the concentration of the photons moving in the beam and as a result radiographic density is affected. It does this because as the focal film distance is changed, the configuration of the beam changes as well. In Figure 87, we see that if an x-ray tube is placed at twenty inches, with the collimator held in a fixed position, a certain field size is achieved. However, if the tube is moved to forty inches F.F.D., diverging photons allow an increased field size. The reason lies in the fact that x-rays travel from the x-ray tube in straight but diverging angles. If the technical factors were held constant,

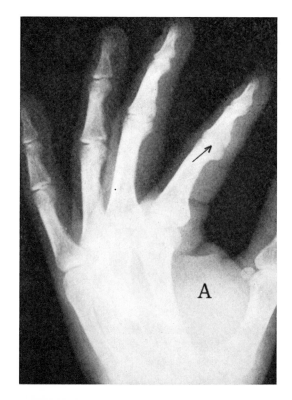

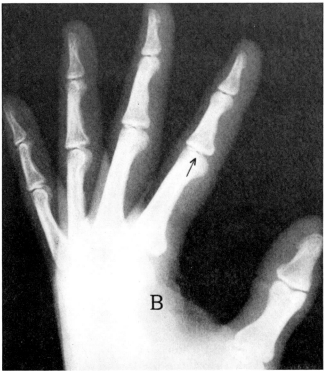

Figure 86. The geometric pattern of the beam requires the technologist to position the tube so the central ray (CR) passes through the body part properly. Angulation or decentering will "close" a joint on the radiograph.

there would be a marked reduction in the density of the image because the same number of x-rays are exposing a much larger area. The net effect of this is that x-ray photons are considerably less concentrated when they reach the film, which results in less ionization of the film's silver bromide crystals over a prescribed area of film.

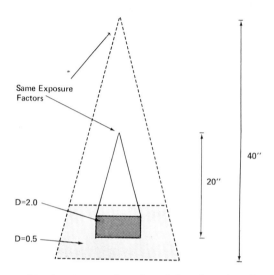

Figure 87. Radiographic density can be altered by changing the F.F.D., because as the focal distance is increased, the *same* quantity of primary radiation is spread over a larger area. The size of the area increases to the square of the distance and radiographic density changes proportionately.

This concept of the same number of x-rays covering larger or smaller areas of film as the result of changes in focal film distance can be expressed in a mathematical formula which tells precisely what the intensity of the beam will be as the focal film distance is changed:

New Beam Intensity = (Original F.F.D.)² ÷ (New F.F.D.)² × Original Intensity

Example: If the original beam intensity is 5r min and the F.F.D. is thirty inches, what would be the beam intensity if the F.F.D. was increased to sixty inches?

$$30^2 \div 60^2 \times 5 = 1.25$$

Example: If the original beam intensity is 10r min and the F.F.D. is fifty inches, what would be the beam intensity if the F.F.D. was decreased to twenty-five inches?

$$50^2 \div 25^2 \times 10 = 40$$

This indicates that the beam's intensity will decrease with increased focal film distance. The technologist must be able to determine the extent of the decrease in order to determine the effect this change will have on the radiographic image. For example, if a given set of exposure factors (MaS and KvP) is used with a twenty-inch focal film distance, the beam's intensity might be 2r per hour. If the F.F.D. is changed to forty inches, it can be determined from the formula that the beam's intensity will be ½r per hour. As a result of this decrease in beam intensity, there would be a corresponding decrease in radiographic density and the technologist must then increase his other exposure factors accordingly to regain the lost density.

The Inverse Square Law is stated as follows: The intensity of the beam is inversely proportional to the square of the distance. Very simply stated, if the focal film distance is doubled, the intensity of the beam will be reduced to one-quarter, as will be the density of the image. On the other hand, if the focal film distance is halved, the intensity of the beam as it reaches the film will be four times greater and the radiographic density will be increased approximately four times. The approximation is made here because the type of film used, as was stated in Chapter Two, affects how it will respond to changes in beam intensity. Figure 88 shows three radiographs using the same technical factors but different focal film distances. Because focal film distance has such a strong influence on radiographic density it can easily be seen why it is considered to be a prime radiographic factor.

FOCAL FILM DISTANCE AND RADIOGRAPHIC CONTRAST

It would be helpful to reflect for a moment on what has been said regarding radiographic contrast. First, radiographic contrast is *not* determined by the *amount* of x-rays produced in the x-ray tube but, rather, by their penetrating ability in combination with the different absorbing properties of the body part under examination (and the ratio of scatter to primary rays exposing the film). Considering the fact that focal film distance does nothing to the beam that would cause changes in penetrating ability, focal film distance would have no effect on radiographic contrast. It might be thought that focal film distance has an influence on the production of scatter and thus would have a strong influence on fog and radiographic contrast. Fog caused by scatter radiation is determined by the ratio of scatter to primary rays *in* the remnant beam and focal film distance has no effect on that ratio.

Choosing the Correct Focal Film Distance

Longer focal film distances will produce a radiograph with better sharpness. However, if too long a focal film distance is used, technical problems would result because other exposure factors would have to be adjusted to compensate for the loss in radiographic density. It has been pointed

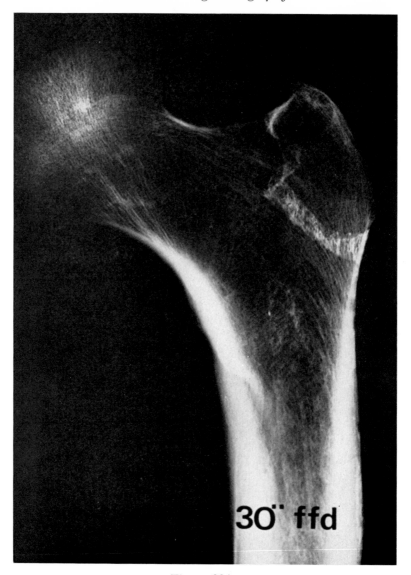

Figure 88A.

Figure 88. These radiographs show the dramatic effect that changes in F.F.D. have on radiographic density.

out that changes in focal film distance cause obvious changes in radiographic density, so a long focal film distance would require a significantly greater exposure to maintain the original density. The increase in exposure could be accomplished by one of three methods: (1) increased Kv; (2) increased Ma; and (3) increased exposure time.

If KvP is increased, there would undoubtedly be a change in radio-

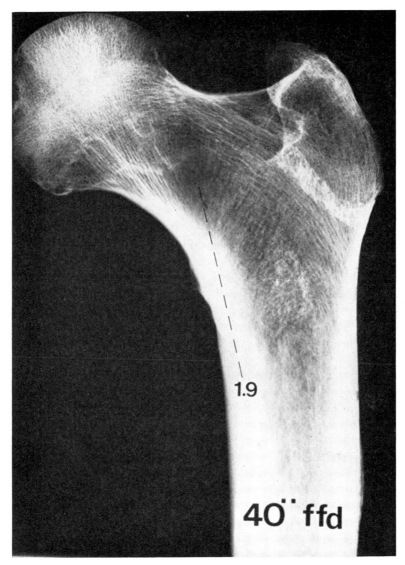

Figure 88B.

graphic contrast which might not be beneficial to the overall radiographic image. If exposure time is increased, the exposure would probably be so long that unsharpness would result from patient motion. If Ma is increased to compensate for increased focal film distance, the life of the x-ray tube might be put in jeopardy because of an overheated anode. For these reasons, focal film distance should be kept constant whenever possible. In the end, the bucky assembly has proved to be an important determining factor in establishing the appropriate focal film distance for most general

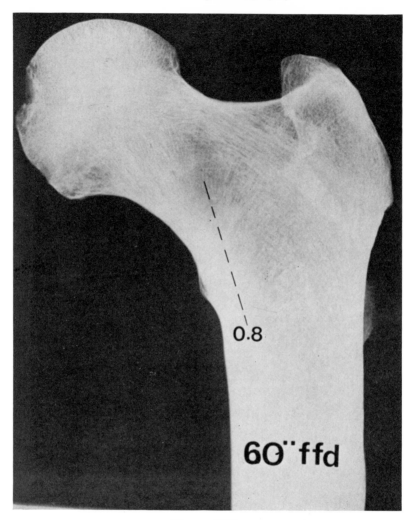

0.8

60" ffd

Figure 88C.

radiography. There is an air space of approximately 2 to 2.5 inches between the patient and the film. This space is needed for various thicknesses of cassettes and for the bucky to work properly, and a forty inch F.F.D. helps to reduce the unsharpness caused by the patient's distance from the film.

In addition to the effect focal film distance has on radiographic density, there is another factor in the geometric image which is very much affected by changes in target distance. As will be seen later, adjustments in the focal film distance has an effect on the sharpness of the various structures in the radiographic image. As focal film distance increases, sharpness or definition of detail increases; short F.F.D. exposures would result in decreased radiographic sharpness.

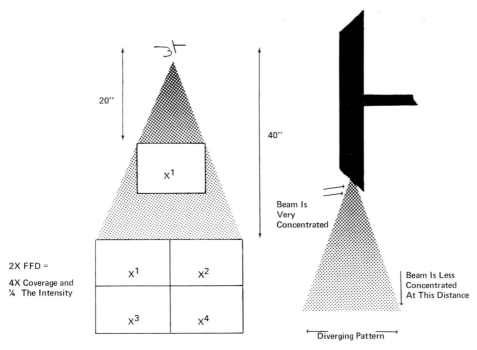

Figure 88D.

THE LINE FOCUS PRINCIPLE

In Figure 89 it can be seen that if a moderately large focal spot is used but is set at an extremely high angle from the horizontal plane, the film *sees* a smaller target area. This is known as *line focus principle* and is an inherent characteristic of all diagnostic radiographic x-ray tubes. In Figure 89, we see the differentiation between the actual focal spot and the effective focal spot. The actual focal spot is a reference to the actual area emitting x-ray photons and the effective focal spot is the area seen by the film. This inherent characteristic of the x-ray tube is basically advantageous for the technologist because it allows use of a larger target area of the x-ray tube, while a smaller focal spot is projected toward the film. When a large exposure is used there is, of course, more heat generated at the target. Unless this heat can be dispersed quickly, the anode of the x-ray tube will begin to crack and become permanently damaged. The use of larger focal spot sizes allows the tube to dissipate the heat away from the target more quickly, thereby decreasing the possibility of tube damage. Also a larger focal spot will permit the space charge to strike a greater area of the target reducing heat intensity over any one area.

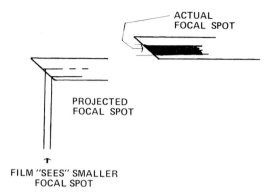

Figure 89. The line focus principle is the relationship between the size of physical focal spots and the size of the projected focal spot seen by the film.

The Point Source

An imaginary type of focal spot is known as the *point source*. A point source refers to an imaginary *point* on the anode from which x-rays might be emitted. For reasons involving tube heat loading, such a target is not possible in practical radiography, but it does serve nicely to illustrate an important concept regarding image sharpness and focal spot size. If an exposure was made with a point source, the projected beam would be slightly different when compared to one that was produced with a focal spot. Specifically, all of the x-rays would be emitted from one tiny spot, whereas with the focal spot or target x-rays would be emitted from all points along its surface (see Fig. 90). When using a focal spot, there are many points of origin for the x-ray photons, and as a result, the beam is composed of many photons criss-crossing each other as they move toward the film and through the body part under examination.

Contrasted with this is the beam produced by the point source, which is *clean* geometrically. In Figure 90, an object has been placed in the beam's path. The resulting image is known as an umbra; this is an ideal situation because there is no criss-crossing of individual photons, so a perfectly sharp image results. However, a focal area, not a point source, is used in radiography, and x-rays are emitted from many points of origin along the target. Under these conditions a notable decrease in sharpness occurs which is known as penumbra. The presence of a penumbra gives evidence that the *entire image* is unsharp. There is always some penumbra present in the radiographic image because of the many x-ray emission points from the target area; however, it can be properly controlled by using the smallest focal spot possible. A comment should be made from a practical point of view regarding this topic. It appears that the effect focal spot size has on radiographic sharpness is limited by the type of

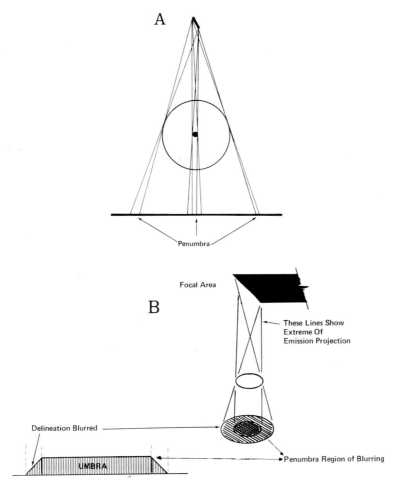

A

Penumbra

Focal Area

B

These Lines Show
Extreme Of
Emission Projection

Delineation Blurred

UMBRA

Penumbra Region of Blurring

Figure 90. A, although a focal spot is the basic cause of penumbra, it must be used to reduce tube loading. B shows poor sharpness which is always present with commonly used focal spot sizes. This unsharpness is present throughout the entire image and not *just* at the penumbra.

screen used. It has been the author's experience that no clearly observable difference in sharpness occurs between large and small focal spots until detail screens are used. Thus, it seems changing focal spot sizes for the sake of showing recognizable improvements in sharpness, while using fast screens, is pointless and even counter-productive considering the increased heat load on the x-ray tube.

As noted a certain amount of object film distance, in addition to screens, causes more unsharpness. Thus, when one asks what effect focal spot size has on sharpness, the answer must be it has a limited effect depending on the type of screens used.

Focal Spot Size

In a practical sense, the focal spot size possesses an interesting problem to the technologist. Small focal spots produce sharper geometric images than larger focal spots, but larger focal spots can withstand a greater heat load which is a very important factor in tube life. Figure 91 shows the same x-ray tube's exposure capacity for various focal spot sizes. Generally, all radiographic x-ray tubes have two focal spots which are usually in the range of from 0.5 mm to 2.0 mm. Newer x-ray tubes, however, are being constantly developed so that smaller focal spots can be used without great fear of damaging the anode. The first of these developments was to change the metal used for the target itself, so it has increased resistance to heat. The x-ray tube is made of tungsten; however, it is coated with other substances that allow quicker heat dissipation than would tungsten alone.

Another advancement in x-ray tube design is the development of the high speed anode. Typically, a high speed anode turns at approximately 8,000 to 10,000 RPM, as opposed to the standard speed anode that rotates at approximately 3,000 RPM. The faster anodes have the effect of spreading the heat generated during the exposure over a greater area, thereby allowing greater heat dissipation and cooling. This is important when very high exposures are made singularly, and especially important when serial exposures are made. When heat loading becomes an especially serious problem, air or water cooled tubes can also be installed which have a definite advantage by increasing the tube loading capacity.

Three Ways to Control Penumbra

Penumbra is the area of unsharpness around the structure in the radiographic image. Figure 92 shows three ways in which penumbra can be controlled: (1) by reducing focal spot size; (2) by increasing focal film distance; (3) by reducing object film distance. Object film distance is the distance between the film surface and the object under examination. The use of a small focal spot size is important where small structures are being examined such as in mammography and various other types of special procedure work. The reason for this is that if the focal spot is larger than the object under examination, *that structure* will become less visible because of extreme penumbra (see Fig. 93).

Because of anode heat problems, manufacturers of x-ray tubes have been very concerned about making focal spots for special purposes as small as 0.3 mm. However, their use is considered by many radiologists to be absolutely essential in such special examinations as magnification techniques. Some extend this 0.3 mm prerequisite to include skull work and tomographic work as well. Here again options should be carefully con-

SINGLE RADIOGRAPHIC EXPOSURE RATINGS

SINGLE PHASE — FULL WAVE RECTIFICATION
STANDARD SPEED (60 Hertz)

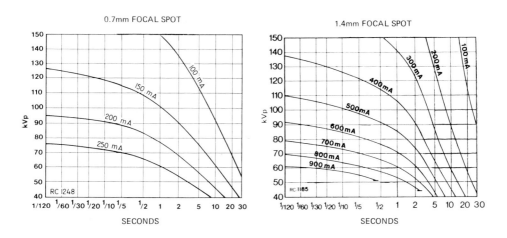

HIGH SPEED (180 Hertz)

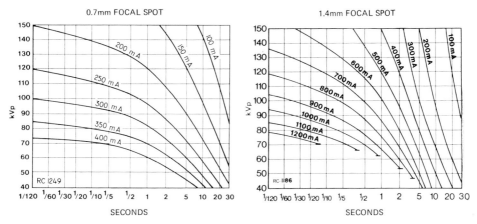

Figure 91. The technologist should know the anode speed, phasing (single or three phase), and the focal size of the tube being used before consulting a tube rating chart. *Courtesy of* Picker X-Ray Corporation.

sidered as small focal spots used with tomography could cause serious tube loading problems, especially with multidirectional tomography.

Figure 94 shows the difference in sharpness between a 2.0 mm focal spot and a 1.0 mm focal spot. In reviewing Figure 120, you will note that the effect of the focal spot size plays a more important role when the object film distance is increased.

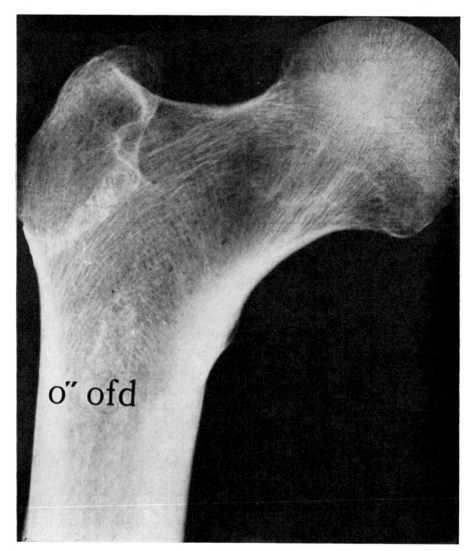

Figure 92A. (40″ ffd)

Figure 92. As the F.F.D. increases from 40 to 80 inches, sharpness improves even when using a larger focal spot.

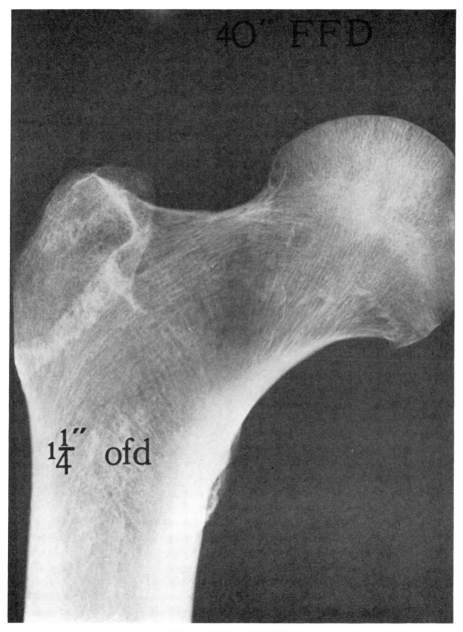

Figure 92B. (40″ ffd)

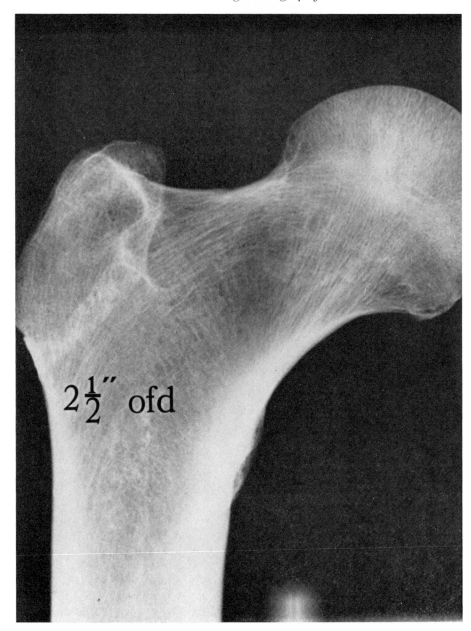

Figure 92C. (40″ ffd)

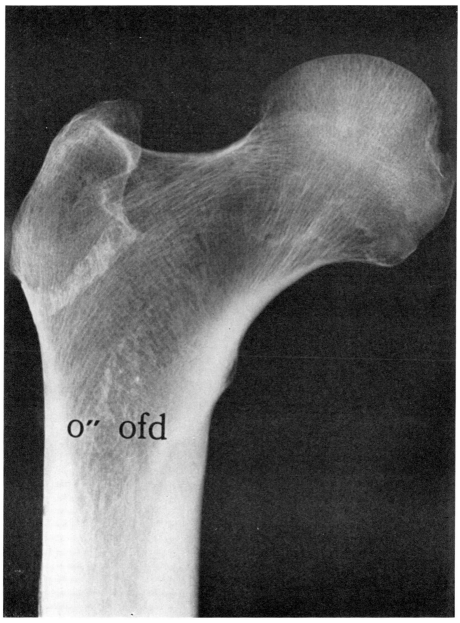

Figure 92D. (80″ ffd)

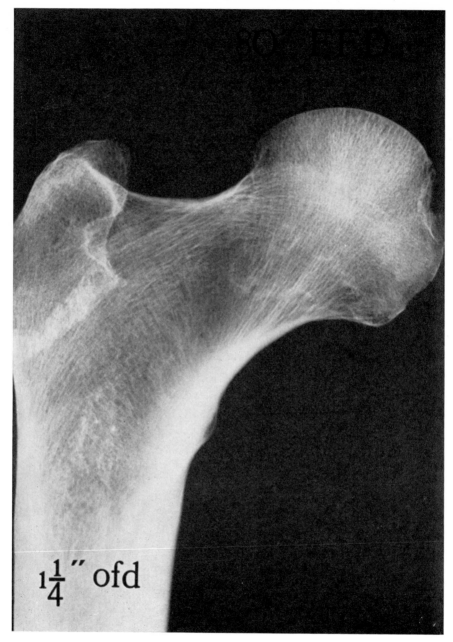

Figure 92E. (80″ ffd)

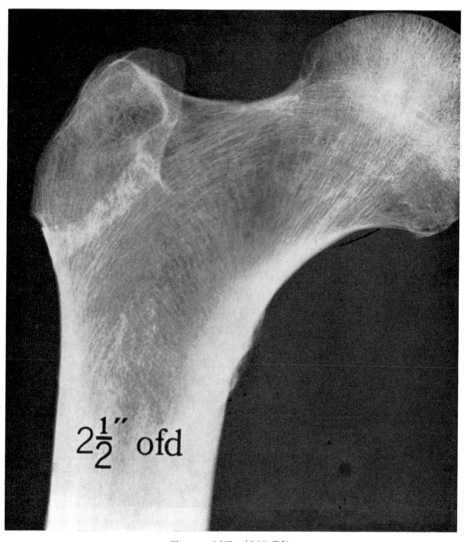

Figure 92F. (80″ ffd)

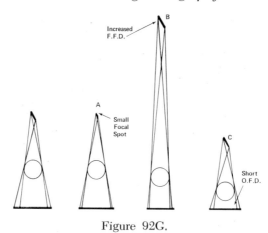

Figure 92G.

OBJECT FILM DISTANCE AND MAGNIFICATION

Object film distance (O.F.D.) must be kept to a minimum. In Figure 95 it can be seen that object film distance plays no minor role in its effect on the geometric image and the resulting radiographic sharpness. In general radiography, there is a necessity for at least a 2.5-inch O.F.D. so that the bucky assembly can work properly. As object film distance increases, penumbra increases. The reason for this is that O.F.D. causes enlargment or magnification of the image which makes the unsharpness more visible, and also the criss-crossing pattern of the beam is greater. Thus, increases in O.F.D. increase the combined effect of enlargement and beam cross-over so body structures become considerably more blurred. It is important to note also that magnification itself is not necessarily a negative aspect in radiology. It might seem so at first, because whenever magnification is produced without taking special precautions, a great deal of unsharpness and blurring results. It is not the enlargement or magnification per se that causes the unsharpness, it is the focal spot or target *area*. Magnifica-

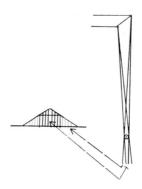

Figure 93.

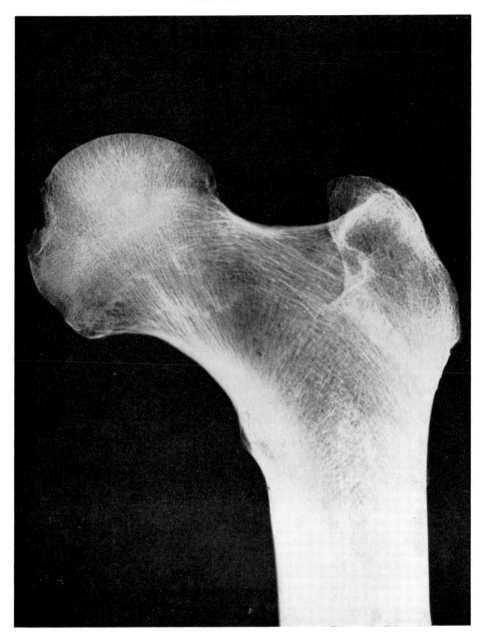

Figure 94A.

Figure 94. The effect of a small focal spot in improving sharpness is more obvious when there is at least a 2 inch object film distance. Otherwise, screen unsharpness has a more dominant role in affecting radiographic sharpness.

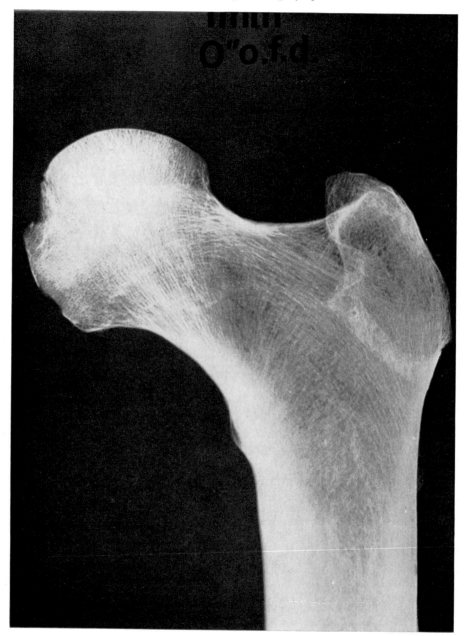

Figure 94B.

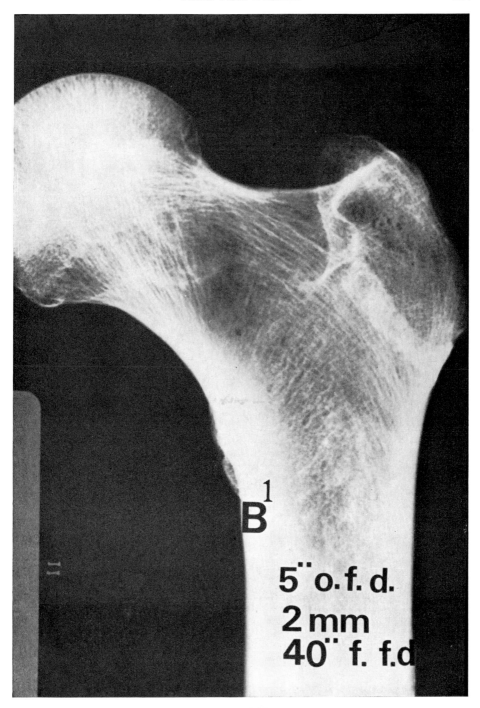

Figure 94C.

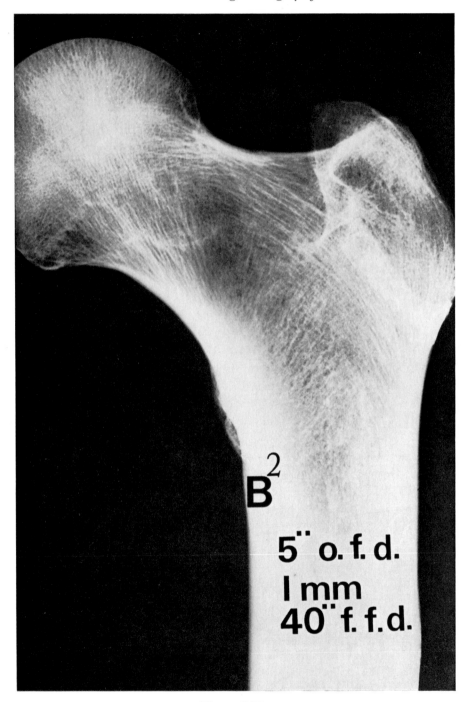

Figure 94D.

tion simply makes the existing penumbra more obvious. Magnification studies are used very often to show tiny but very important structures that might otherwise have gone unnoticed; when using magnification work, a fractional focal spot size is essential.

Common studies are performed when the location of a specific body part gives rise to a kind of inherent object film distance because of its location in the body. Thus, it is important to know that the body itself can often produce object film distance on its own. Occasionally, more than the usual 40 inch focal film distance is required to produce good radiographic sharpness of these body parts. In such an instance the body can be obliqued or rotated so that the immediate structure under examination is at the closest possible distance to the film. When the technologist comes upon a situation in which the object film distance of the body under examination cannot be changed by rotating the patient, the focal film distance should be increased. An example of this is the lateral cervical spine film. If the patient is in the lateral position and the film is touching the shoulder there is approximately a 6 inch object film distance, and if the focal film distance was not changed, magnification and decreased sharpness would result in the various structures of the cervical spine vertebral bodies. As a result of this, lateral cervical spine films are routinely done at 72 inches. Making spot films of a lateral thoracic and lumbar spine using 48 inch focal film distance would improve the radiographic sharpness of the vertebral bodies. Of course, when the focal film distance is increased in this way adjustments in the other exposure factors must be made to maintain radiographic density.

In summary, unnecessary object film distance should generally be avoided whenever possible because it usually results in decreased sharpness and in magnification which makes the unsharp structures more obvious. The technologist should increase focal film distance whenever possible to compensate for object film distance.

The Magnification Technique

Because radiologists have become accustomed to the present size of the various body parts as seen in the radiographic image and considering that one of the most important indicators leading to a roentgen diagnosis is the proper evaluation of structure size, there is some reluctance in using a magnification technique. However, the magnification technique has proven to be an important asset in roentgen diagnosis. This method is simply known as the magnification technique and it is most commonly employed while doing special studies involving vascular opacification. Cullinan and others, for some time, have advocated its use and laid important groundwork for its technical development and improvement. In Figure 96, you will see an examination of a renal arteriogram comparing conventional and magnification technique. Very little imagination is required to see the advantage this procedure offers when viewing small, complex vascular configurations.

Prerequisite for Magnification Technique

The primary prerequisite for accomplishing good magnification work lies in the use of what is known as a fractional focal spot. You will recall from the previous discussion that using a smaller focal spot increases radiographic sharpness. With magnification technique, the object film distance is varied to obtain the desired degree of enlargement. If the object under examination is located at the midpoint between the tube and the film, the resulting image will be approximately two times greater than the actual body part. The potential danger in doing magnification work is that the very small focal spot sizes required have very poor heat loading characteristics because of the tremendous heat concentrated on the relatively small target area. With this in mind the technologist must be extremely careful to choose exposure factors that will not exceed the tube limits of a single exposure or a rapid series of exposures. A second problem common to magnification technique is in centering the beam correctly. One should be able to imagine how a longer object film distance would affect the possibilities of having the image centered on the

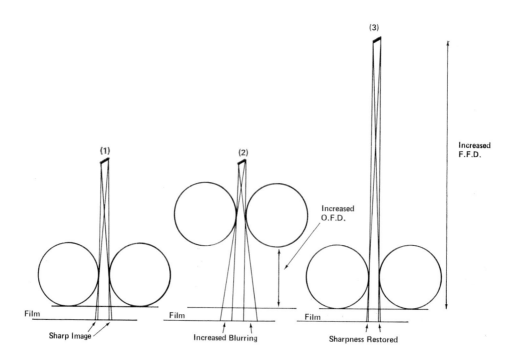

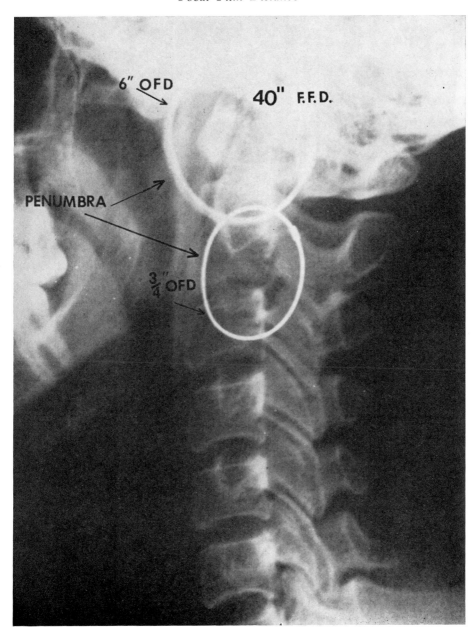

← Figure 95. Object film distance does not "cause" penumbra while focal area does. Increased O.F.D. enlarges penumbra and makes it more obvious. The root cause of this type of unsharpness is that photons are being emitted from a focal area in opposing tangent planes. The F.F.D. should be increased when possible if a large O.F.D. is present. If the cervical spine had been exposed at 72 inches, the variation in magnification and sharpness between the rings would be greatly diminished.

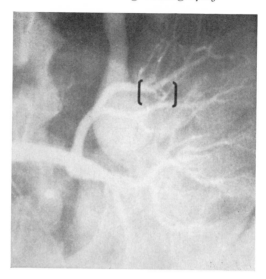

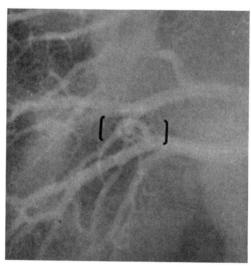

Figure 96. The magnification technique can be more easily appreciated after reviewing these radiographs.

film as the result of the diverging rays. The problem of centering is important in routine radiography, but with magnification technique it becomes crucial. If an object is not placed in the core of the beam but rather among the more divergent angled rays, the image will be shifted laterally to a certain extent. The degree of lateral projection would depend on how far away from the center ray the object is located. With magnification technique a small amount of decentering produces a disproportionate increase of lateral shifting and distortion (as noted in Fig. 97).

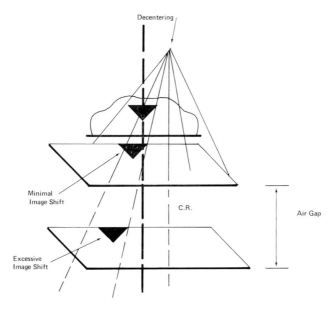

Figure 97. Decentering will be discussed later along with the air gap technique. It is imperative that the CR be centered directly over the body part.

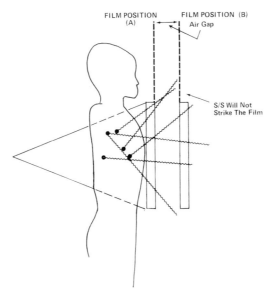

Figure 98. The air gap technique is much less effective when higher KvP levels are used, because scatter photons travel more directly toward the film.

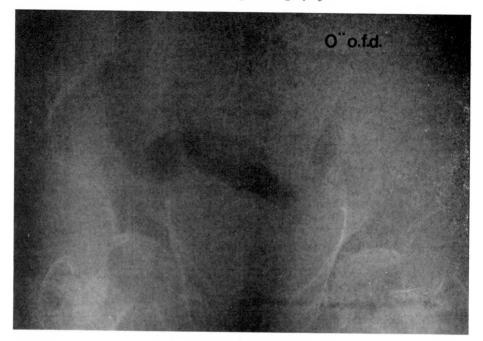

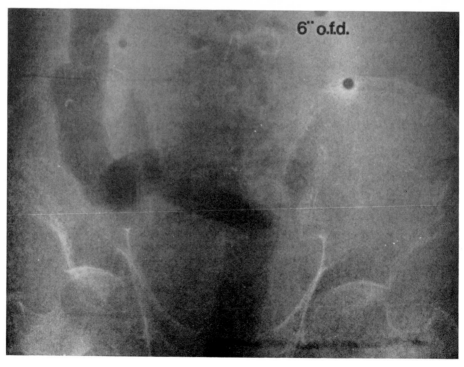

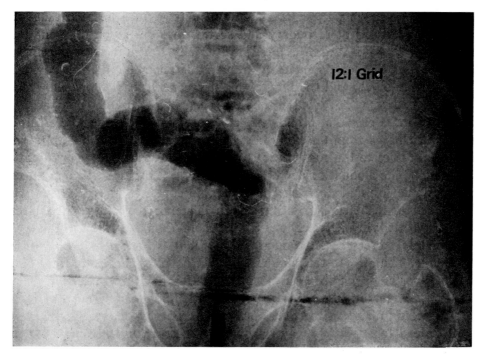

← Figure 99. Pelvis using the air gap technique to demonstrate its effect on the radiographic image. Because of the absence of scatter photons reaching the film, radiographic contrast increases and density decreases. Also shown is a comparison using a 12:1 grid.

In summary, magnification technique is an important tool to have at one's disposal and depending on the radiologist it is something that is not merely an option but essential. The major purpose is to enlarge the image and thus make more visible very tiny body structures that might otherwise go undetected.

Usually, an enlargement factor of 100 percent is used and is achieved by placing the object under examination at midpoint between the film and the x-ray tube. The primary technical problems with doing magnification work are tube loading and decentering. In reference to tube loading the technologist may consider one of the new rare earth type screens and moderately fast film. The rare earth screens fortunately help this problem by allowing a considerably shorter exposure to be used.

Object Film Distance and Scatter Radiation

Although it is important in routine radiography for the object film distance to remain as short as possible, occasionally a long object film distance can be used to the technologist's advantage. If the beam's normal diversion projection pattern is brought to mind, it can be seen that the projection patterns of secondary and scatter rays are much different (as noted in Fig. 98). Because scatter rays usually travel at a greater angle compared to that of the primary photons, if enough space is provided between the object and the film, many of these scatter photons emerging from the body may never reach the film. The primary rays, by comparison, are much more predictable and certainly more direct so we can be assured they will emerge from the body part correctly and will continue to travel in straight lines to the correct area of the film. The reason for our interest in reducing the amount of scatter is, of course, that excess scatter produces radiographic fog and decreased radiographic contrast. Thus, one can see how changes in object film distance can influence the amount of scatter radiation that will ultimately reach the film. When focal film distance is deliberately increased to produce this effect it is known as the air gap technique. The air gap technique requires a definite increase in focal film distance so that penumbra can be controlled. As with magnification technique, improper centering is also a potential problem. The author's feeling regarding air gap procedures is that, considering the problems even well trained technologists may run into with centering large patients for chest examinations, the added inconvenience associated with an object film distance of approximately 10 inches gives the procedure questionable value. Also, although many scatter rays are eliminated from reaching the film, many more could be eliminated with the use of a 10 or 12:1 ratio fine line stationary grid. Figure 99 shows the effect of an air gap with a pelvic examination.

Additional Advantages in Using Increased Object Film Distance

A more effective use of long object film distances is to improve visualization of structures that lie over one another in the body and result in superimposed structures on the film. Such superimposed body parts cause confusing densities in the radiographic image and often make the particular part under examination barely visible. In such instances, object film distance can help the radiologist and technologist. Figure 100 shows an area of the body that possesses this problem and thereby lends itself well to using an increased object film distance. There are other such areas of the body and if the technologist would consider this point for a second these may come to mind. In the meantime, the mandible is an easy and convenient example to consider. With the head in the lateral position one mandible is approximately 6 inches away from the film. With a 40-inch focal film distance, the two mandibles are superimposed making it very difficult to distinguish both structures radiographically. However, if the

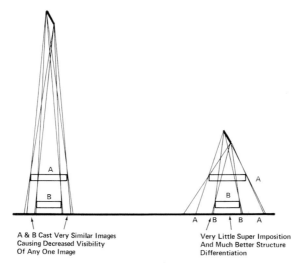

A & B Cast Very Similar Images
Causing Decreased Visibility
Of Any One Image

Very Little Super Imposition
And Much Better Structure
Differentiation

Figure 100.

focal film distance is reduced to 20 inches, the effect of the 6 inch inherent
body object film distance becomes very much exaggerated and produces
an extreme amount of penumbra. With a greatly increased penumbra, the
sharpness of the structures begins to fade slightly as the more sharply defined structures of the body part close to the film become more visible
by comparison. Occasionally technologists have reduced the focal film
distance to the point where the collimator is almost touching the patient's
face. This is successful only when the specific body part under examination
is directly against the cassette. Very often bucky work, because of the
2.5 inch object film distance, is not as successful in producing the desired
effect. In fact, the condyle away from the film is almost invisible because
of the extreme penumbra produced by the combination of increased object
film distance and short focal film distance. The net result of this technical
manipulation of O.F.D. and F.F.D. is to reduce the visibility of the
condyle which is not under examination, thus making the other condyle
more visible. Once again it should be emphasized that the key to success
when using this method is to keep the body part under examination not
close but immediately against the film.

DISTORTION OF THE RADIOGRAPHIC IMAGE

Shape Distortion

Shape distortion occurs when the radiograph shows the object under
examination to be different in form from the actual body part of the

patient. Shape distortion (or true distortion as it is often called) is a condition that occurs automatically when x-rays pass through a body part at an incorrect angle or when the plane of the film is tilted (see Fig. 101). Magnification is a quite different situation than shape distortion. Often it appears that dramatic angulation of the center ray and the film often causes poor radiographic sharpness. However, the actual reason for this is not a result of the angled beam per se but, rather, a result of the increased object film distance that often occurs when the beam is angled (as noted in Fig. 102). It can be seen here that the projected image of the part under examination travels a further distance to the film as the tube is angled, thus producing increased blurring. Occasionally, angulation of the tube is necessary to improve the demonstration of certain body parts. However, if the beam is properly centered, shape distortion will be kept to a minimum. The Towne's view, for example, requires the center ray to be angled at least 30°. The resulting radiographic image gives the skull an oval shape which, of course, is shape distortion. The body parts inferior to the sella turcica seem to stretch endlessly toward the bottom of the film. Because the beam is properly centered, distortion of the body part immediately under examination is kept to a minimum. Tube angulation can also be used to reduce the superimposition of various body parts (as noted in Fig. 103). Here a sigmoid view of the colon made with the tube angled 35° causes an "artificial" straightening of the sigmoid. Many other possibilities can be mentioned here, however, it is sufficient at this point to simply present the idea of angulation of the beam to achieve certain positive results, and alert the reader to be watchful of the negative effect that improper angulation can have with regards to shape distortion.

Size Distortion

Size distortion is frequently used as a synonym for magnification. Size distortion is caused by the fact that x-rays are emitted from the target in increasing divergent angles as they pass through the body and reach the film. Object film distance and focal film distance determine the extent to which magnification or size distortion occurs. It might be helpful to use some examples so the relationship between focal film distance, object film distance, and magnification can be more easily analyzed. It should be understood that there is no standard object film distance or focal film distance that can produce optimal results. Magnification is controlled by the relationship between focal film distance and object film distance. For example, a good radiographic image can be obtained with a 2 inch object film distance and a 40 inch focal film distance, but an equally good image would be obtained if a 4 inch object film distance were used, providing an 80 inch F.F.D. is used. This is an important point to understand because

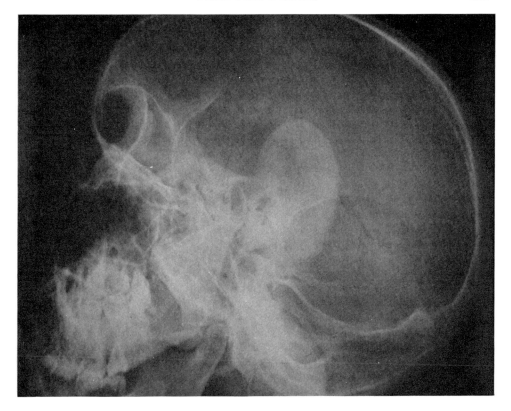

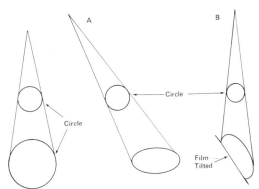

Figure 101. This properly positioned lateral skull is distorted because of faulty tube alignment.

when doing unusual or difficult cases, such as cross-table, operating room, or portable work, placing the body part directly against the film is very often impossible. However, if the technologist keeps in mind that the critical factor for good sharpness and minimal size distortion is to produce a proper relationship between object film distance and focal film distance, a sharp and nondistorted radiograph of the body part can be produced. As noted earlier, when the technologist comes upon a situation where the object film distance may not be or can not be decreased, the focal film distance should automatically be increased. Figure 104 summarizes these concepts.

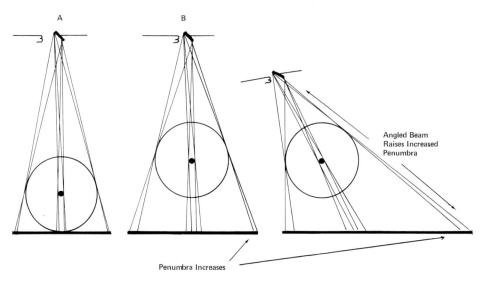

Figure 102. The O.F.D. increases automatically as the tube is angled.

Stereotactic Procedures

There are some occasions where proper centering is required well beyond what is normally achieved in routine radiography. A surgical procedure known as stereotactic demands unusually precise centering and no distortion whatever. The procedure itself involves the placement of a small electrode into the pituitary gland of the brain. This is done by advancing the electrode through a bore hole in the patient's skull and inserting the probe through a very narrow space between the two hemispheres of the brain. It is impossible for a surgeon to know exactly where the electrode is during this procedure without x-ray control. During the procedure, a series of radiographs are thus made to pinpoint the progress and location of the electrode as it is moved through the brain to the pituitary gland. Needless to say, anything less than absolute precise calculation is not acceptable as permanent brain damage could result. Once the electrode is in place, a small electrical charge is placed to the gland with the intention of permanently deadening its activity. Precise centering with zero magnification and shape distortion are characteristics of the stereotactic x-ray procedure.

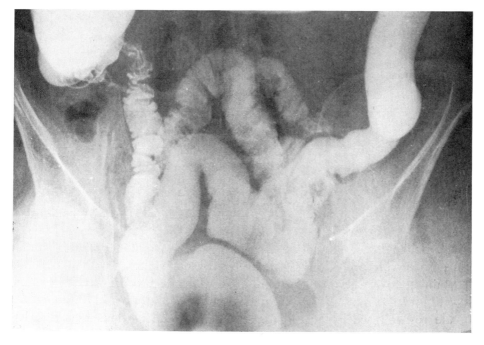

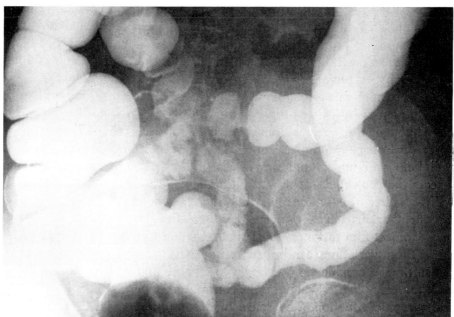

Figure 103. The angled CR makes an area of many superimposed structures more visible.

MAJOR GEOMETRIC FACTORS   RADIOGRAPHIC EFFECT

		Radiographic contrast	Radiographic density	Size Distortion	Shape Distortion	Geometric Unsharpness
F.S.S.	Focal Spot Size					X
F.F.D.	Focal Film Distance		X	X		X
O.F.D.	Object Film Distance	x*	x*	x		X
A.C.R.	Angle of Central Ray				X	

* Only when increased o.f.d. allows scatter radiation to escape and not expose the film.

Figure 104. How the various geometric factors affect the radiographic image.

A pelvimetry examination is also very important geometrically. The purpose of this procedure is to supply the gynecologist with information pertaining to the size of the baby's head relative to the dimensions and position of the mother's birth canal so that a decision can be intelligently made regarding delivery technique. Accurate calculations regarding the degree of magnification are very important here as well. The relative sizes of the baby's head and the mother's birth canal are very important measurements and thus must be radiographed with a minimal amount of distortion using proper centering and positioning of the center ray.

The procedure for radium implant localization is another example of how much the projected image influences the radiographic image. Here, again, measurement calculations are necessary and distortion must be kept to a minimum by using proper centering.

Although the various items discussed in this chapter may at first seem confusing or complex, actually they are not. The illustrations shown will help you understand how each of the geometric factors discussed affects the projected image and ultimately the radiographic image. There are a number of variations in which these factors relate to each other and produce various effects, however, if the basic concepts of focal film distance, object film distance, focal spot size, and tube angulation are kept in mind these variations can be worked out with some individual thought.

In time, a confidence will begin to emerge that will considerably benefit the technologist when he is confronted with a difficult emergency radiographic situation. The sense of accomplishment as a result of performing one of these exams is well worth the initial effort.

The Anode Heel Effect

A chapter covering the projected or geometric image would be incomplete without at least a brief discussion of the anode heel effect. This

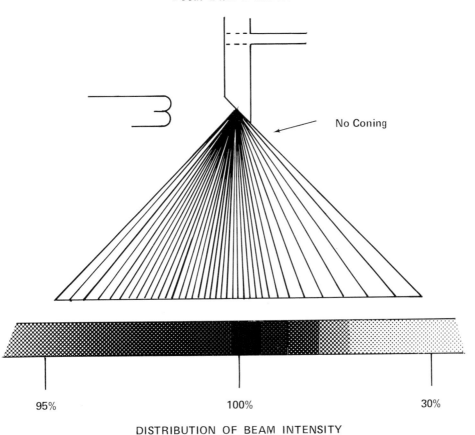

DISTRIBUTION OF BEAM INTENSITY

Figure 105. The variation of beam intensity is primarily at the peripheral edges, not in its core.

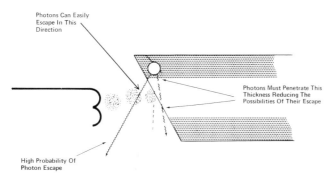

Figure 106. As the newly "born" x-ray photons pass through the thicker portion of the target, fewer are able to escape causing an inconsistency of beam intensity.

area of radiography is so often confused and misused that some clarification needs to be made with regard to its practical application in radiography. This phenomenon of the heel effect is caused by the angle (bevel) of the target. Figure 105 illustrates schematically the anode heel effect as it relates to the variation in intensity along the long axis of the x-ray tube. It should be pointed out that the anode heel effect has little practical influence on the radiographic image. As was pointed out earlier in this chapter, the x-ray beam travels from the target in a divergent pattern with increasing angles from the core of the beam to its perimeters. The extreme changes in beam intensity at the perimeters is the result of partial absorption of the x-ray photon in the anode material itself (see Fig. 106).

It is true that such intensity in beam variations exists; however, you will note that this variation occurs primarily at the outer peripheral rays—during routine radiography an assortment of beam-limiting devices are always used, thereby (see Fig. 107) eliminating these peripheral rays from affecting the radiographic image. If two chest exposures are made, one with the patient's diaphragm under the cathode portion of the tube and the other with the patient's diaphragm under the anode end of the tube, there will be very little difference between them.

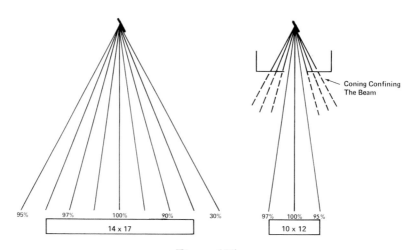

Figure 107.

In summary, the anode heel effect is caused by partial absorption of the x-ray photon by the anode; it should be understood that there are three factors that affect the extent to which this occurs radiographically. One, of course, is the use of beam-limiting devices. As the collimator is closed more tightly, the possibility of an x-ray film experiencing different intensities of the beam is decreased substantially. Second, as the angle of the anode increases from a horizontal plane, the heel effect becomes more exaggerated. The third major factor that influences the anode heel effect is the focal film distance, as shown in Figure 108. As focal film dis-

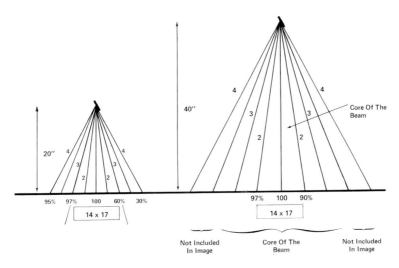

Figure 108.

tance increases, the possibilities of the anode heel effect being seen in the image become considerably decreased because more of the center portion or core of the beam is utilized for the exposure.

CHAPTER SEVEN

KILOVOLTAGE

C HAPTER FIVE described the method by which electrons are produced to form the space charge. The space charge alone would have no value to the technologist if it did not also possess an additional form of energy that could later be converted to x-ray energy. Frequently technologists feel that it is the electron itself that undergoes the conversion process into x-radiation. Instead, it would be more correct to say that the electrons making up the space charge are simply vehicles upon which kinetic energy rides to the anode. The electrons collide with the anode but then pass through the anode into the high tension circuit and past the Ma meter. We will discuss in this chapter why kilovoltage, an electrical term, is so important to the technologist in producing a radiographic image.

DEFINITION AND FUNCTION

Kilovoltage is electrical pressure caused by an abundant supply of electrons at one side of the circuit. It is the nature of this imbalance to "want" to become balanced. This "need" manifests itself in a situation where the electrons at the oversupplied (negative) side of the circuit will begin to move toward the deficient side to effect the balance (see Fig. 109). When one electrode with a very strong negative (−) charge is placed near a second electrode with a positive (+) charge, there is a natural tendency for these charges to attract each other and eventually equalize or balance. The electrical pressure that was caused by the inequity between the two electrodes causes electrons to flow, and in so doing, current is registered. The level of kilovoltage in the circuit is determined by the degree of imbalance between these charges, and as the electrical imbalance of the charges increases, electrical pressure would likewise increase. This would result in greater voltage (faster moving electrons through the circuit). The voltage will continue as long as there is an electrical imbalance, but as soon as the imbalance of charges is equalized, the voltage will drop to zero and the electrons, of course, will stop moving. This concept is relevant to radiography because the technologist uses

[174]

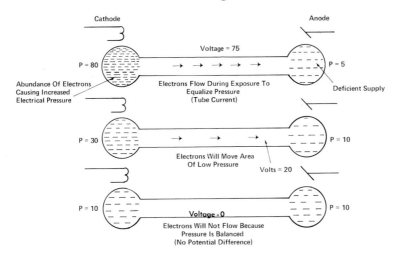

Figure 109. The speed of electrons moving from cathode to anode is dependent on the imbalance of electrons in the x-ray tube.

KvP to set up various levels of electrical pressures within the x-ray tube. This in turn has a very strong effect on the quantity and quality of x-ray photons that will ultimately be produced. It is a common misconception that Ma is the only factor that influences the total quantity of primary radiation, however, it has been well documented that KvP plays an important role in determining the quantity of primary radiation in a given x-ray exposure as well.

Kilovoltage, Tube Current, and the X-Ray Tube

As you read through this chapter, many important factors will be discussed. However, they will all be totally dependent upon the influence Kv imposes on tube current. In order to produce an x-ray beam, three criteria must be met: (1) A supply of electrons is needed; (2) they must be given a high level of kinetic energy; and (3) the electrons must be suddenly stopped thus converting their kinetic energy into radiation.

The supply of electrons, of course, forms at the filament of the x-ray tube as a result of filament heating (see Fig. 110). These electrons (in the tube) act as vehicles upon which kinetic energy rides. Earlier, it was said that uneven or imbalanced charges seek to balance themselves. The x-ray tube has two electrodes known as the cathode and the anode. Under normal conditions, the cathode has the negative (—) charge, which means it has an abundant supply of electrons, and the anode has a positive (+) charge, which means that it has a deficient amount of electrons; under these conditions, electrons will begin to flow from the cathode toward the anode. X-rays are produced when the electrons of the tube current strike and interact with the atoms of the anode.

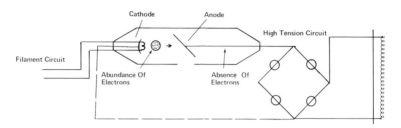

Figure 110.

To explain the process of how kinetic energy is converted into x-radiation, an analogy of an automobile collision has some application. If we observe an automobile moving at the speed of ten miles per hour and it collides with a stone wall, a transformation or conversion of energy will result. The kinetic energy built up by the motion of the car suddenly becomes nonexistent when the car reaches the wall and is stopped. Under the law of conversion of energy, something must happen to that kinetic energy, because "energy cannot be created nor destroyed." What actually occurs is that the kinetic energy transforms into heat and sound waves. If we observe the same type of car moving with a higher level of kinetic energy of 40 miles per hour, the higher level of kinetic energy built up in the increased speed would be transformed into a higher level of heat and sound.

A similar kind of energy conversion takes place in the x-ray tube as the kilovoltage is raised and lowered to control the speed of tube current. It should be pointed out that the car functioned as tube current does in carrying kinetic energy. However, the kinetic energy in the x-ray tube is converted into heat and x-radiation. The x-ray tube then is simply a device used to convert kinetic energy into x-ray energy, but it is very inefficient because up to 99.8 percent of the kinetic energy of the tube current becomes heat and only 0.2 percent is eventually converted to x-radiation. The x-radiation emitted by the anode in this conversion process is known as primary radiation (see Fig. 111). It should be noted that the *actual percentages* will increase or decrease as different KvP levels are used; however, it has been generally held that 0.2 percent is a fairly accurate figure to use for discussion purposes.

In summary, this discussion can be outlined as follows: X-rays are formed when a high level of kinetic energy is achieved by the space charge in traveling from the cathode to the anode. This radiant energy is of a high frequency (short wavelength) and the specific level of the kinetic energy of the tube current is, of course, dependent upon the kilo-

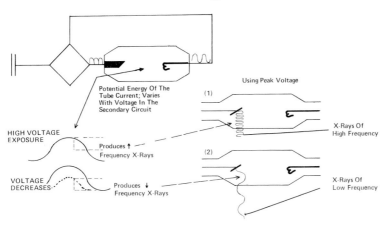

Figure 111. Whether high or low energy x-rays are produced, interactions between the anode and the space charge cause primary radiation. As tube voltage increases, more efficient conversion takes place and a higher primary beam is produced.

voltage set by the technologist before the exposure is made. The higher the kilovoltage used, the greater the electrical pressure will be between the cathode and anode, and the faster the electrons will move toward the anode. This will cause greater quantities of primary x-rays and greater x-ray energy (penetrating power).

KvP = ↟ Kinetic energy = ↟ Conversion Numbers = ↟ Energy of x-ray photons

Kilovoltage and the X-Ray Circuit

It is important that we draw some concepts regarding how the electrical pressure is generated in the x-ray tube. Figure 112 shows a very simplified drawing of an x-ray circuit. We will begin at the primary circuit where the incoming current is taken from a main 220 volt supply. The autotransformer is responsible for adjusting this incoming voltage to achieve higher or lower kilovoltages. It does this by using a series of "taps" that are directly connected to the KvP selector located on the x-ray control panel. The selected voltage passes through the primary circuit to the high tension transformer where it is boosted approximately 500 times its previous value. If the autotransformer produces a voltage of 100 on the primary side of the circuit, it will become 50,000 volts after it reaches the secondary of the high tension transformer.

Figure 112 shows the relationship between the high tension transformer, the cathode, and the anode. It can be seen that, when a technologist chooses a high KvP setting, an electrical pressure is set up accordingly in the tube. It can also be seen from the illustration how the x-ray tube actually bridges the connections between the filament circuit and the high tension circuit. During the exposure, the filament circuit

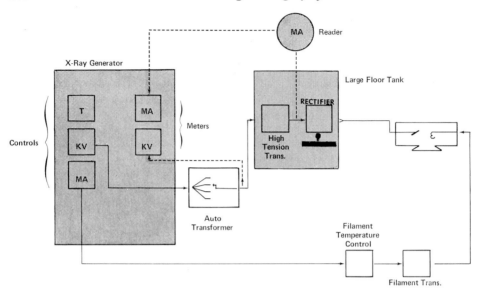

Figure 112.

produces the space charge which is then driven toward the anode by the high voltage.

BEAM QUANTITY AND QUALITY

If one considers *primary radiation* as possessing two separate aspects or characteristics, it will be easier to understand the concepts of beam quantity and quality. Further, if the technologist can gain an understanding of how these characteristics can be adjusted and balanced in each exposure, he will have gone a long way toward becoming a competent radiographic technologist. One can correctly say that, under normal working conditions, a radiographic image is very dependent on the balance between quantity and quality of radiation produced and, as was pointed out earlier, the KvP chosen by the technologist for a given exposure has a great deal of influence on both these beam characteristics. As was noted earlier, KvP was traditionally not thought of as playing a significant role in affecting the quantity of x-ray photons produced at the anode; however, this myth should be discarded, but this certainly does not deny the very strong effect MaS has on beam quantity. However, MaS does not *exclusively* control beam quantity. This can be summarized in the statement below:

$$\text{KvP} = \frac{\text{Beam Quality}}{\text{Beam Quantity}} = \frac{\text{Radiographic Contrast}}{\text{Radiographic Density}}$$
$$\text{MaS} = \text{Beam Quantity} = \text{Radiographic Density}$$

Kilovoltage and Beam Quality

An x-ray photon can have various penetrating abilities depending on the KvP. A low KvP exposure will produce x-ray photons with relatively low penetrating abilities, and a high KvP exposure will produce a beam with higher energy and penetrating abilities. If all other factors are held constant, as KvP increases, more photons will penetrate the patient and make a darker image. Penetrating ability, beam quality, and beam energy are terms that are synonymous. The terms wavelength and frequency can be confusing. Figure 113 shows two x-ray beams: As the frequency increases, wavelength decreases.

Wavelength Distribution

The x-ray beam is made up of rays known as photons or quanta. In a normal diagnostic exposure, these individual *packets of radiant energy* (quanta) vary from one another in their individual frequency (see Fig. 71). For example, if the technologist chooses 80 KvP at the control panel, a wavelength of perhaps 0.3 angstroms will be predominant, but the beam will also contain photons ranging in wavelength from several angstroms to a minimum of 0.155 angstroms. Each diagnostic exposure has some variation in wavelength, but they do make up a "common" identifiable beam. If an x-ray beam contained photons that were very much different from each other with regard to frequency, the term heterogenic, poly-

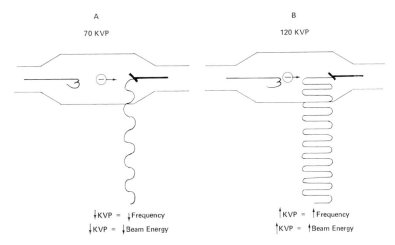

A
70 KVP

B
120 KVP

↓KVP = ↓Frequency
↓KVP = ↓Beam Energy

↑KVP = ↑Frequency
↑KVP = ↑Beam Energy

Figure 113. Increases in KvP produce a beam with overall greater frequency (energy) x-ray photons even though not all of these primary photons are equal in frequency. These gray scales demonstrate the effect KvP has on contrast (the same objects were used in all cases shown). As the KvP was increased, the objects' parts experienced different absorption rates with respect to each other, altering subject contrast and ultimately radiographic contrast.

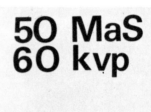

**50 kvp
25 MaS**

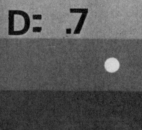

Figure 113A.   Figure 113B.

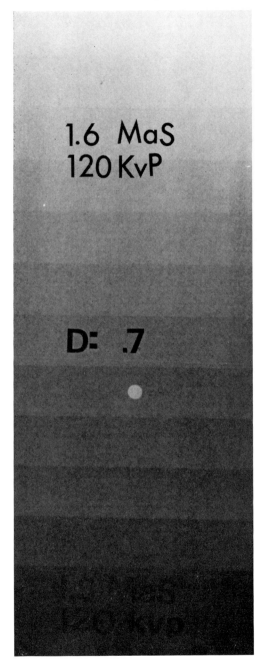

Figure 113C.

chromatic, or polyenergetic would apply. However, if another beam were emitted from an x-ray tube that contained photons with the same frequencies (equal penetrating power) the term homogenic or monoenergetic beam would apply. This is an extremely important concept because the predominance of high or low energy photons in a beam almost totally influences subject contrast and, ultimately, radiographic contrast. The thickness of filtration also influences the mixture of photons in a given beam.

KILOVOLTAGE AND SUBJECT CONTRAST

Controlling subject contrast is absolutely vital to good radiography, and the main factor used to control subject is kilovoltage. Subject contrast exists when two or more body parts absorb x-ray photons differently. Figure 114 illustrates the radiographic effect of subject contrast. As was mentioned earlier, the body has a complex arrangement of absorbing tissues and structures. Indeed, the body has characteristic "regions" of subject contrast, such as the chest, abdomen, extremities, and the skull.

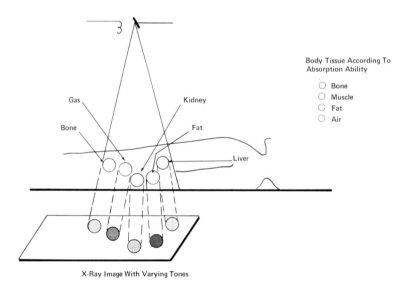

Figure 114. Some of the absorption differences in the body.

The chest exhibits the ability to absorb x-ray photons differently and, accordingly, it is often referred to as a high subject contrast region. The abdominal region, however, is something quite different because its individual body parts are composed in such a way that they absorb the beam much more uniformly and, understandably, this region is known as a low subject contrast area. As will be discussed later in the text, one of the

most important steps the technologist must take in producing a high quality radiograph is to know how to adjust KvP so the beam exiting the body
(remnant radiation) will produce the best possible image. The remnant
beam will be given special attention in Chapter Eleven, but a brief discussion is required here to show its relationship between subject contrast
and the radiographic image.

In order to explain subject contrast, we will use the example of a
stained glass window made with pieces of variously sized and colored
glass. These variously colored pieces of glass *individually* allow only so
much outside light to pass through. The observer is actually experiencing
how these opposing *dark-* and *light-*colored sections are absorbing the
sun's light to cause different degrees of light intensity. The observer's eyes
sense these wide *variations* in *light intensities.*

In Figure 115, we can imagine that one glass section is made with
similar light-absorbing abilities, such as light green, light blue, and beige;
these *similar* colors will absorb the sunlight uniformly, causing low subject contrast. In a section of window with an arrangement of sharply con-
trasting colors of glass, the sunlight is absorbed by the individual pieces
of glass with greater variance, and we perceive this as having a high subject contrast.

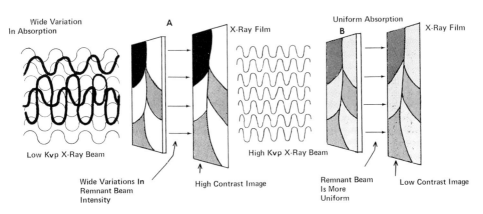

Figure 115. The primary x-ray photons vary in their absorption, resulting in subject
contrast. Subject contrast is affected by the characteristics of the body and the energy
of photons attempting to pass through.

The various body parts also allow x-ray photons to penetrate and be
absorbed. If a body region contains structures that absorb the beam at
widely varying degrees, the remnant photons emerging from the body
part will have widely varying intensities and, as a result, will cause corresponding densities on the x-ray film producing a radiograph with high
contrast. A lower subject contrast would result if individual structures

produced a remnant beam with somewhat uniform intensities (resulting in a more uniform density pattern on the film's emulsion).

Later, we will discover more about why different body parts have different absorbing abilities; however, for now it is important that we understand that the beam's ability to pass through the body is controlled by the technologist as he manipulates KvP. These two factors determine whether or not the intensities of the remnant beam will be uniform. Thus, the degree of variation or uniformity in the intensities of the remnant beam will ultimately affect the degree of radiographic contrast. This important concept is outlined in the two statements below:

> (A) High KvP exposures result in photons of higher energy, yielding uniform penetration and producing films with low subject contrast and low radiographic contrast.
>
> (B) Low KvP exposures result in photons of lower energy, yielding a variance in penetration of body tissues and producing films with high subject contrast and high radiographic contrast.

EXPOSURE LATITUDE AND KILOVOLTAGE

The word latitude, in general, is a term that tells the degree of acceptance or tolerance. When exposure latitude is used in a radiologic sense, it tells to what extent an exposure can be changed before the diagnostic quality of the image is threatened. In other words, exposure latitude tells how much an exposure can be altered before a noticeable change results in diagnostic value. Kilovoltage has a unique effect over exposure latitude, as you will see in the following example. If an exposure was made at 60 KvP, an increase to 69 KvP should approximately double the radiographic density over what was obtained with 60 KvP. If, however, the *initial* KvP was 110, an increase of 16 would be necessary to achieve the same radiographic effect. Because of this, it is said that KvP influences exposure latitude (see Fig. 116). As KvP increases, exposure latitude widens or increases as noted in this example. With this in mind, it can be seen that there are some advantages to using high KvP exposures. In general when high KvP techniques are used, technique adjustments become less critical. However, there are two side effects associated with high KvP exposures (100 KvP and over) that are not necessarily advantageous.

1. As KvP increases, additional scattered photons reaching the film can cause fogging.
2. Often the body parts under examination have a very low inherent subject contrast; when a beam is used that penetrates that part too uniformly, subject contrast becomes too low, producing low radiographic contrast.

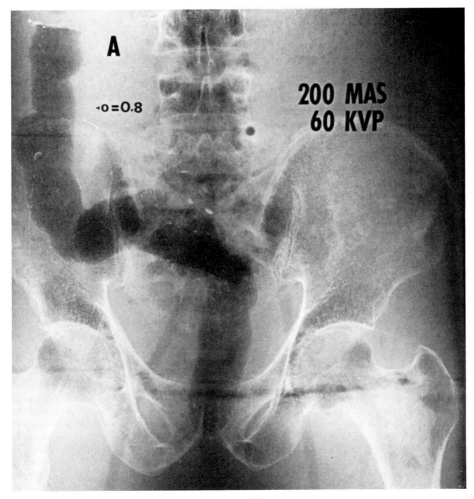

Figure 116A.

Figure 116. Similar density changes have resulted between *A* and *B* and between *C* and *D*: A 9 KvP increase in the 60 KvP range produced approximately the same density changes (*A* and *B*) as a 16 KvP increase in the 110 KvP range (*C* and *D*).

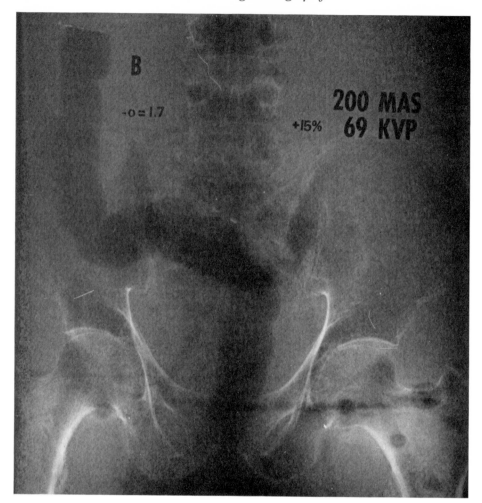

Figure 116B.

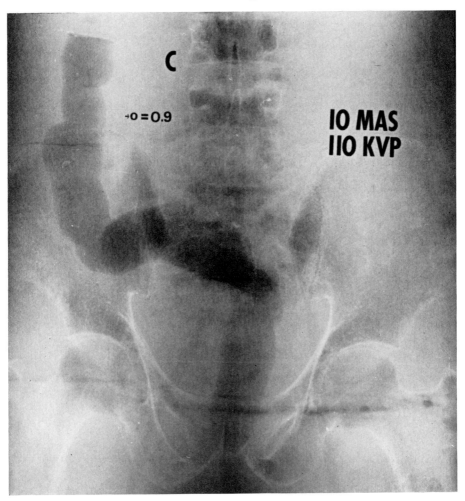

Figure 116C.

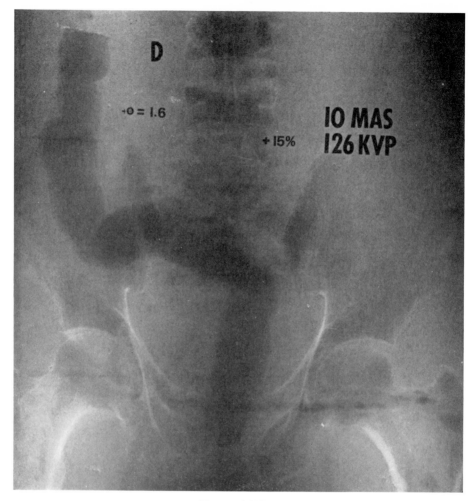

Figure 116D.

Kilovoltage, Patient Dose, and Beam Efficiency

Not only does KvP have a strong effect on the radiographic image, it affects the patient dose as well. As we know, the body has great variation in structure, which causes the beam to have more or less difficulty in penetrating the body while en route to the film. As an x-ray photon passes through the patient, it will undergo one of the following: (a) total penetration; (b) total absorption; (c) partial absorption. (See Fig. 117.) The type and number of interactions produced in the body during an exposure has an effect on the quality of the image as well as patient dose. The level of KvP used for each exposure determines, to a large extent, which of the resulting interactions will be dominant. A high KvP setting, for example, will produce a higher level energy conversion at the anode

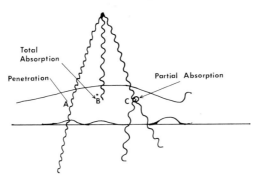

Figure 117: The *type* of photon-tissue interactions that result during an x-ray exposure is greatly affected by the energies of the individual photons—which are controlled by KvP.

and will, in turn, produce a more penetrating beam. With such an exposure, fewer numbers of photons are needed to obtain the same density and result in an overall lower patient dose. A lower KvP exposure, on the other hand, will produce a lower energy conversion at the anode and the beam's penetrating ability will be greatly diminished as more absorption type interactions are likely to occur. If a beam of low penetrating energy were to be used, a greater quantity of radiation would have to be produced to assure sufficient radiographic density. Thus, beam efficiency is an important concept for the technologist to keep in mind when formulating x-ray exposure factors: As KvP increases, beam efficiency increases and patient dose decreases (Fig. 118 illustrates this point). The first condition noted in this figure indicates comparable radiographic density is achieved with less patient dose and less tube current. Keep in mind that when less tube current is used, as seen here, the anode can operate at a lower heat

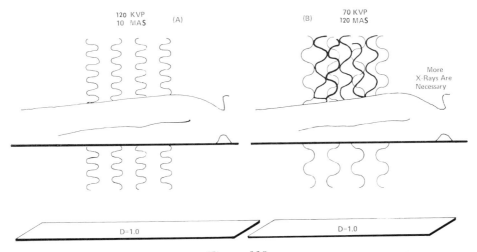

Figure 118.

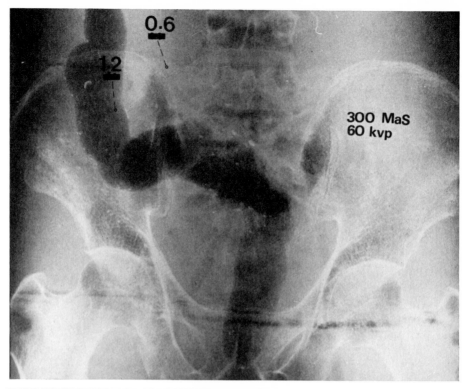

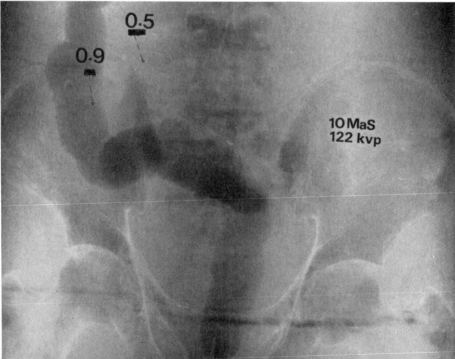

Figure 119. The effect KvP has on subject and radiographic contrast is indicated by the actual densities shown. Observe the MaS values necessary to produce similar densities when the KvP is changed. Also the densities shown indicate changes in contrast.

level which enhances its life expectancy. With this, one can correctly say that kilovoltage levels have an influence on patient dose by virtue of their effect on beam efficiency. If higher KvPs are used, fewer x-ray photons are needed to produce the same radiographic density. Figure 119 shows radiographs that have been exposed with high KvP and low MaS compared with low KvP and high MaS exposures.

KILOVOLTAGE AND SCATTER PRODUCTION

Diagnostic exposures cause secondary radiation. However, for practical purposes, the energy of secondary photons produced in a typical diagnostic exposure have no effect on the radiographic image. On the other hand, scatter production is very influential over the appearance and diagnostic value of the radiographic image. The total amount of scatter production is dependent on a number of factors. Although they will not be discussed completely until Chapters Eight and Nine, it is appropriate that they be listed here. As long as the amount of filtration is held constant, the five items below will control the total amount of scatter radiation produced in a given diagnostic exposure.

1. Tissue density
2. Thickness of tissue
3. Atomic number
4. KvP level
5. Field size

Between the two extreme cases of total penetration and total x-ray absorption, the intermediate case of partial absorption (or scatter production) exists. One may correctly say that scatter rays are a type of "by-product" that if not controlled will cause radiographic fog. When one realizes that up to 90 percent of the x-rays reaching the film during an exposure of an abdomen are scattered rays, one can more realistically appreciate how important it is to choose the proper level of KvP in order to prevent an excessive amount of scatter production. Although there is scatter production present in all x-ray exposures, it must be kept in mind that radiographic contrast does not necessarily deteriorate due to large quantities of scatter, but rather because of an imbalance in the ratio of scatter to the number of primary photons that strike the film. The proper ratio of scattered to primary photons in the remnant beam must be maintained for good radiographic quality to result.

When the ratio of scatter to primary photons is out of balance, radiographic fog results. Figure 120 illustrates this important concept. The term scatter ratio, of course, refers to the relative amounts of scatter and primary photons that are present in the remnant beam. The most im-

portant type of interaction producing large amounts of scatter in the diagnostic exposure is known as the Compton interaction: As kilovoltage increases beyond 70 the relative numbers of Compton interactions produced
in a given exposure increase substantially. In other words, as the KvP increases over 70 scattering type interactions are more common when compared to the total absorption type, known as photoelectric interactions,
and will result in a condition known as scatter fog (which greatly reduces radiographic contrast and visibility of detail by producing an additional veil of density over the radiographic image).

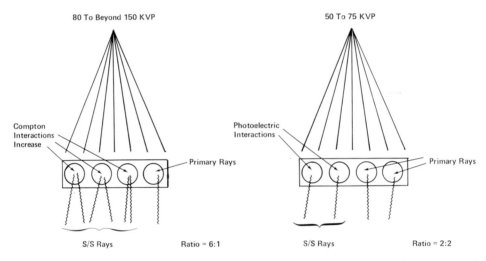

Figure 120. As the quantity of scattered photons increases relative to the quantity of
primary radiation, the possibility of fog increases dramatically. The figures used are
hypothetical.

There is another phenomenon that occurs with high KvP exposures
which increases the likelihood of scattered rays reaching the film. With
lower KvP exposures, the scattered rays travel in greatly divergent angles
as compared to the primary photons. Because the scattered photons are
so divergent in direction many do not reach the film. However, as higher
KvP values are used for a given exposure, the scattered rays produced
tend to move in a more direct line toward the x-ray film. The result of
this, of course, is that the film experiences a greater exposure by scattered
rays and the probability of fog increases. Also, these more direct scattered photons have greater penetrating ability, causing even more scattered photons to reach the film with predictable results on the radiographic
image.

Thus, kilovoltage has a tremendous effect on radiographic contrast
because of its control on scatter production and its effect on subject con-

trast. Lower kilovoltages produce more of the total absorption type of interactions in the body (commonly known as the photoelectric effect). This type of interaction is much more sensitive to differences in tissue composition, i.e. tissues with varying atomic numbers and densities. It should be pointed out further that this type of interaction, although it may produce a radiographic image with higher contrast, also produces an increase in total patient dose. Thus, once again, a kind of trade-off must be made between the type of radiographic contrast desired and patient dose when establishing a technique chart.

After reading through the material in this chapter, one might have the impression that it is generally a good practice to lower the kilovoltage to control the relative amount of scatter and increase subject contrast. Before any such changes are made one must carefully consider that kilovoltage is the only prime factor we have available that controls the penetrating ability of the beam, and if it is lowered too much, the body part will not be penetrated adequately (see Fig. 121). KvP levels should be set to primarily establish proper contrast and adequate penetration of the part being examined, and then be left alone using MaS to regulate radiographic density. The method used to control scatter should be left to the use of proper coning and proper selection of grid ratio.

Base KvP is a term that is used to describe the least amount of KvP that will provide adequate penetration for a particular body part. Although the base KvP does not apply perfectly for every radiographic condition, it is generally an adequate guide and will serve the technologist well in arriving at a valid starting point for establishing new exposure factors.

$$\text{Base KvP} = \text{body part thickness in cm} \times 2 + 30 \text{ KvP}$$

Since the average KvP applied across the x-ray tube is greater with three phase equipment, lower KvP settings will be required: To find base KvP for three-phase equipment, it would be more correct to add 20 KvP instead of 30.

Kilovoltage, Radiographic Density, and Contrast

No mention has been made, up to this point, specifically regarding KvP and radiographic density. We already know that, if the milliamperage is raised, the quantity of primary photons being emitted by the anode is raised by roughly the same proportions and radiographic density increases. If KvP is increased from 70 to 80, the second exposure will produce approximately twice the density. Thus kilovoltage does have an effect on radiographic density, caused by the fact that KvP produces more energetic photons which will more easily pass through the body. Also as KvP increases, the number of primary photons increase as well because more

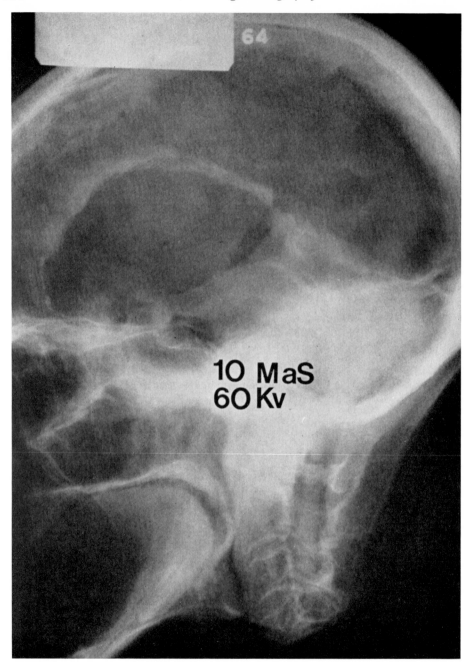

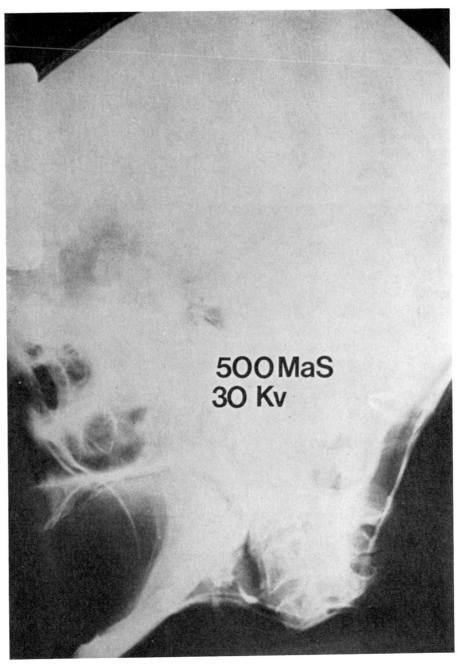

500 MaS
30 Kv

← Figure 121. If the KvP is lowered too much for a particular body part, no practical increase in MaS will produce a diagnostic image.

efficient conversion occurs from the tube current's kinetic energy into
x-rays.

Radiographic contrast is the difference between two tones or densities.
For example, if density "A" is 2.0 and density "B" is 1.0, the contrast between the two is 1. If density "C" is 0.5 and "D" is 0.75, there is a 33 percent change in density if we measure "C" against "D". However, if we
wanted to measure "D" against "C", the value would be 50 percent.

As was pointed out above, KvP influences radiographic contrast as a
result of its effect on the subject. Recall the description of the stained
glass window: The eyes responded to the glass pieces that absorbed the
sun's light as radiographic film responds to the varying intensities of the
x-rays passing through the body. In one area there was uniform light
penetration and, as a result, variation in light intensity was low, yielding
a low contrast image. In the other section of the stained glass, the light
penetrated nonuniformly. In this instance, a high contrast situation existed
which was transferred to the film. In a sense, the x-ray film "sees" and
records these various intensities of the remnant beam (see Fig. 115).

An IVP examination is illustrated in Figure 122. The area of the opacified kidney and those structures immediately adjacent to it demonstrate
a high subject contrast. Note how this changes as the kilovoltage is increased. Lower KvP exposures produce a predominant number of total
absorption type interactions (photoelectric) that are very sensitive to body
parts with respect to their varying atomic numbers and tissue densities.
This can be seen in the statements below:

> (1) Decreased KvP produces increased numbers of total absorption inter-
> actions, yielding increased subject contrast and increased radiographic contrast
> (also less scatter).
> (2) Increased KvP produces increased partial absorption interactions, yield-
> ing more uniform penetration of body parts and decreased subject contrast
> (also increased scatter production and decreased radiographic contrast).

From the statements above and by reviewing Figure 122, we can begin
to see how KvP levels should be chosen for a particular body part. When
radiographing a body part with a high inherent subject contrast, low
KvP chest exposures probably would yield excessive radiographic contrast.
Chest examinations lend themselves well to high KvP exposures. Also,
because the chest region contains a large amount of air along with low
density lung tissue, scatter production can be controlled very readily by
using a high ratio grid. When radiographing an abdomen, it would be
wise to use a lower KvP; this would produce more total absorption versus
total penetration type interactions, and greater variation in tissue absorption would result. Subject contrast would increase and scatter production
would be kept to a minimum as well. The net result of this would be
higher radiographic contrast with better visibility.

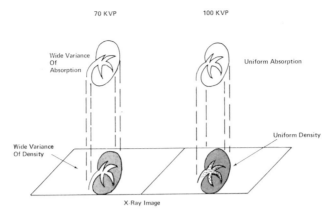

Figure 122. Since many absorption interactions are present in a low KvP exposure, the contrast medium in the kidneys allows fewer x-rays to reach the film, producing a higher radiographic contrast.

In summary, it can be said that the body is composed of very complex structures with many different absorption properties and it behooves the technologist to appreciate how the various beam characteristics (frequency and type of interaction) affect subject contrast and ultimately radiographic contrast (see Fig. 123). With this knowledge the correct choice of KvP can be made.

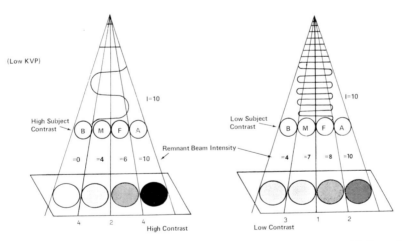

Figure 123. Radiographic image is dependent on subject contrast (differential absorption).

Fixed versus Variable KvP Techniques

With the mass of information discussed thus far, only a few final observations need to be made regarding KvP. One of these is how a technique chart can be written; there are two basic systems commonly used today: (a) optimum or fixed KvP and (b) variable KvP. A fixed KvP technique chart is one in which the KvP level is held constant for all thicknesses of a given body part. Abdomens, for example, might be exposed at a 75 KvP regardless of the measurement. Of course, some compensation is necessary for various thicknesses and MaS is used to serve the purpose for adjusting radiographic density. Most often, the exposure time is adjusted to compensate for patient thickness. In general, the KvP initially chosen for each body part must meet some prerequisites to insure against underpenetration. Also, it is important to choose a KvP that will provide optimal radiographic contrast, as noted earlier. To help establish the proper level of KvP the five criteria listed below should be examined:

1. Ability of the body part to absorb the primary beam.
   a. tissue density
   b. atomic number of the tissue
   c. tissue thickness
2. Inherent subject contrast versus the type of radiographic contrast scale desired.
3. The ability of the body to produce S/S.
4. Grid ratio available.
5. Special examinations where subject contrast must be enhanced or possibly de-emphasized, i.e. chest work, injected contrast media, mammography.

A fixed KvP technique chart does have some important advantages. In short, the major advantage in maintaining consistent KvP for each body thickness is that radiographic contrast tends to be more consistent. A disadvantage of optimal or fixed KvP is, of course, exposure time is increased with body thickness resulting in the possibility of increased patient motion. The principle of fixed KvP technique is used in all manufacturers' phototimed equipment. When a phototiming system is used, the technologist selects the proper KvP and the automatic phototimer changes the exposure time according to the patient. Because of the serious limitations that high milliamperage exposures have on tube loading, it is generally considered that varying the Ma to compensate for body thickness and radiographic density is a very poor practice. If a sufficient number of Ma stations were made available, this disadvantage could be eliminated or greatly reduced and the problem of excessively long exposure times would be eliminated.

With variable KvP techniques, a KvP is chosen for an average thickness of a body part. This is often a subjective choice made in accordance with the criteria listed earlier. The kilovoltage is then increased or decreased according to body thickness as the milliamperage and time factors are held constant. Figure 124 shows an illustration of both the variable and fixed Kv type methods. Note that with a variable KvP chart, the

	FIXED KvP							VARIABLE KvP						
ABDOMEN A.P.	CM	Kv	Time	Ma	Grid	F.F.D.	Scn	CM	Kv	Time	Ma	Grid	F.F.D.	Scn
	17-18	80	2/10	300	12:1	40″	Fast	17-18	80	2/10	300	12:1	40″	Fast
	19-20	80	3/10	300	″	″	″	19-20	84	2/10	300	″	″	″
	21-22	80	4/10	300	″	″	″	21-22	90	2/10	300	″	″	″
	23-24	80	1/2	300	″	″	″	23-24	96	2/10	300	″	″	″
	25-26	80	7/10	300	″	″	″	25-26	102	2/10	300	″	″	″
	27-28	80	9/10	300	″	″	″	27-28	108	2/10	300	″	″	″

Figure 124. The relative techniques (for an abdomen, fast screens, slow film) needed for variable and fixed KvP methods.

KvP is increased by increments of two for every cm of patient thickness. As was pointed out earlier, time and Ma do not change, so relatively short exposures can be used regardless of part thickness. However, because of the effect that Kv has on exposure latitude, thicker body parts require higher KvPs and so greater increases than two Kv are required per cm thickness. For example, if a knee measuring 12 cm requires 70 KvP, a second knee measuring 13 cm would require 72 KvP. If the KvP level were 95 for the 12 cm knee, a knee measuring 13 cm would require 100 KvP. The major problem with variable KvP charts is that radiographic contrast is not consistent. As higher KvPs are used, subject contrast decreases and the degree of S/S fog often increases. A fixed KvP technique chart using high KvP exposures is accepted in modern radiography and would have the advantage of decreased patient dose as well as shorter exposure time.

CHAPTER EIGHT

THE HUMAN BODY AS AN EMITTER AND BEAM
MODIFIER

THE MANY CONCEPTS presented thus far are extremely important to good radiographic quality. Yet one important item has not been considered: the human body. Its complexity and function are matched only by its variation in form and absorption characteristics, and it is these variations that can cause technical havoc for the technologist. When we think of a tall, lean individual, a certain body form comes to mind; this type of body form (habitus) can produce a great number of different x-ray absorption rates that, if understood, will make it much easier for the technologist to choose correct exposure factors. Such body variations can come in the form of an abdominal obstruction, cardiac enlargement, evacuation of air from the lungs, atrophy of bone and soft tissues, and many other possibilities. Figure 125 demonstrates an assortment of these pathologic problems; the reader should notice how they vary from normal body composition.

Recently, the use of automatic timing devices has helped considerably in making automated exposure adjustments for radiographing such maladies, and this trend will probably continue. Even with phototiming, the technologist must have a sound working knowledge of how the body modifies the primary beam into a series of intensities that ultimately expose the film's emulsion. With this introduction to the "patient problem," it is certainly no understatement to say the human body is by far the single greatest variable in radiography. Often technologists can develop a type of intuition that will serve them well in making the final decision in favor of one specific set of exposure factors as opposed to another. With some practical understanding of how body habitus relates to radiography, the technologist will eventually be able to *predict* with confidence how he can alter the primary beam via exposure factors to produce the desired radiographic result. A seasoned technologist can almost "see" how the beam will pass through the body part under examination and imagine the beam as it is absorbed differently by the internal structures, *before* the exposure is even made. In short, no matter how accurate or complete a

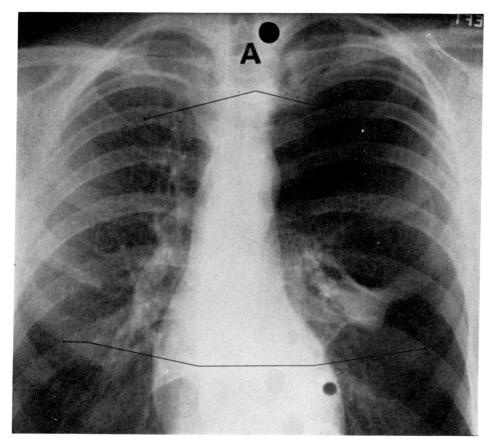

Figure 125A. A dramatic change in appearance between the right and left side of the chest due to a collapsed left lung.

technique chart may be, the technologist is responsible for making the final adjustments to achieve optimal diagnostic results.

MAJOR ABSORBERS OF THE BODY

Fortunately, humans do have some basic similarities in composition. The major substances that account for most of the x-ray absorption are fat, fluid, muscle, and bone. Equally sized fat globules from one patient will be equal in absorption to that from another person, and the other four body substances are also equal from one to another person. The *distribution* and *quantity* of these are usually responsible for the confusion when choosing the correct set of exposure factors for a given patient.

Another aspect that can weigh heavily in formulating a technique is the presence of air in the body. As with the other major body components, its presence alone is often not as important as how much there is. In short,

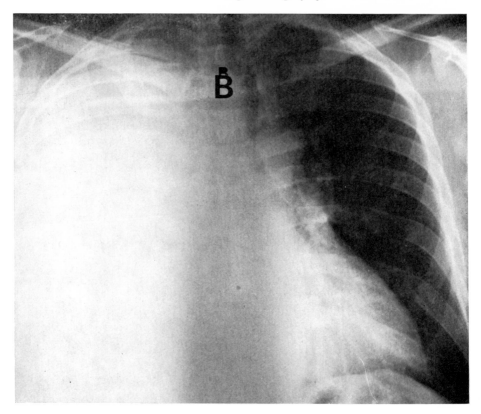

Figure 125B. The entire right side of the chest is filled with fluid; it is difficult to penetrate the chest with this type of pathology.

the technologist can more effectively manage the situation at hand by "technically pigeonholing" the patient as to (1) the quantity and distribution of the major tissues being radiographed, (2) age of the patient, (3) the pathology that might be present within the patient, and (4) how the primary beam may be altered (what interactions will take place) by these various characteristics. In the remainder of this chapter we will attempt to point out how all these body aspects both hinder and help the technologist and offer some suggestions for making the problem more manageable.

Some General Facts Regarding Body Habitus

The body is made up of approximately 62 percent water, 15 percent fat, and 23 percent bone; approximately 40 percent of the total body weight is muscle (at age seventeen). Of the soft tissue substances, muscle has the greatest water content and this has an important bearing on the radiographic image. Fat contains less water as compared to muscle tissue.

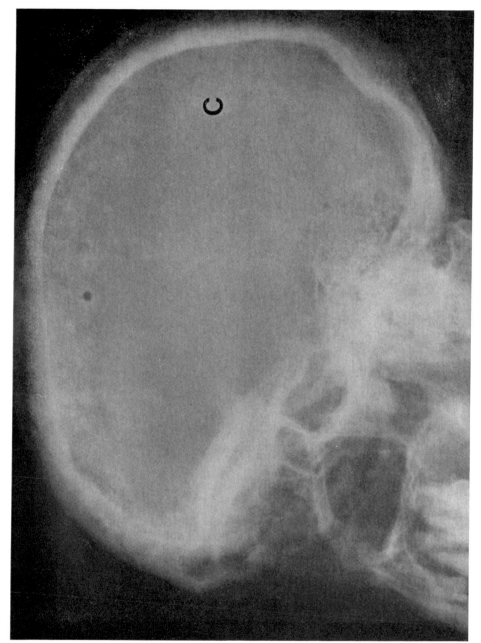

Figure 125C. A skull revealing a condition known as Paget's disease where the bone becomes quite dense and difficult to penetrate.

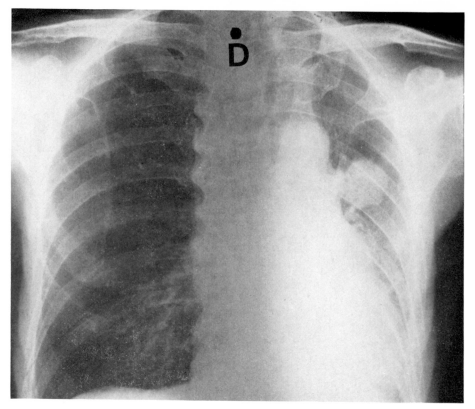

Figure 125D. A totally collapsed left lower lobe, secondary to bronchogenic Ca.

Body fluid itself is more absorbent to x-rays than muscle tissue. Healthy bone absorbs more x-ray photons than body fluids, fat, or muscle; however, the greatest absorbing substance in the human body is tooth enamel.

Fat Content

As noted above, when fat is compared to muscle it has a lower water content and slightly different atomic number. It should be kept in mind that water is extremely efficient in producing scatter radiation. As noted earlier, the water content alone will have an important effect on the radiographic image. Large amounts of muscle tissue would produce more scatter than an equal amount of fat, and thus muscle is likely to cause a considerable decrease in radiographic contrast. Radiographic density will also decrease because muscle absorbs more photons than fat. There is no doubt about the deleterious effect S/S fog has on radiographic contrast. It is interesting to note that most technologists expect to see a decrease in radiographic contrast resulting from radiographing fat people. A typical image that results when radiographing a fat patient is increased

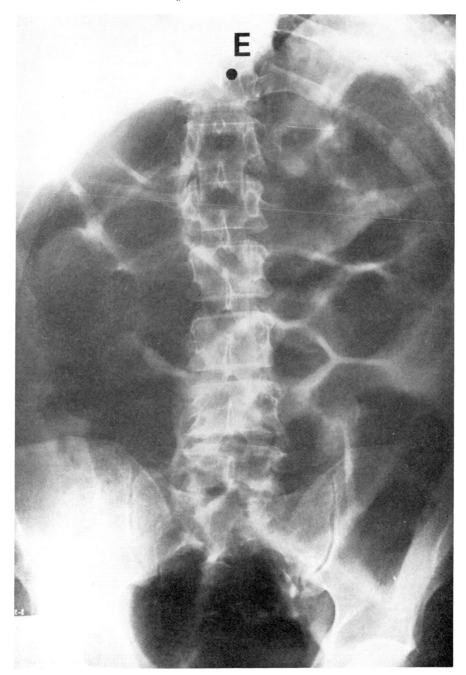

Figure 125E. An abdomen distended with air.

density with a gray, flat appearance. The explanation for this lies in the fact that when obese patients are radiographed, the organs themselves are encapsulated amidst thick fatty layers which generally reduce the relative differences in x-ray absorption between the organs and the tissues immediately surrounding. Thus, obese patients simply have much less subject contrast and Figure 126 schematically demonstrates this concept.

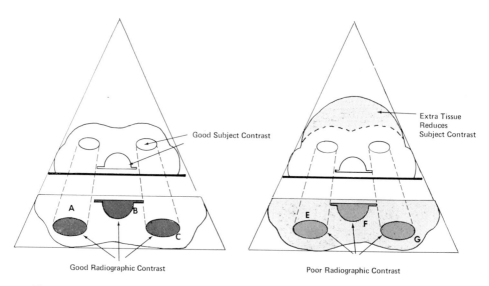

Figure 126. The additional fatty layer causes a reduction in subject contrast.

Also, if carefully analyzed, a radiograph of an obese patient may be poor in quality simply because the film has been over-exposed. Fat is not very absorbent to x-rays, i.e. if two large patients measuring approximately the same were radiographed using the same exposure factors, the fatter patient could produce a darker image. With this in mind, one should consider how technique factors might be chosen for obese patients. Many times the technologist, because of patient size, becomes slightly intimidated and thus has a tendency to simply overexpose the radiograph. Often the technologist would obtain a better radiographic image of such a patient if the technique were actually reduced slightly, preferably with KvP; this would cause a moderate to obvious increase in subject contrast. The author has seen many obese patients, measuring as much as 28 cm for an A-P abdomen, done very successfully with 70 KvP. Figure 127 shows two radiographs of the same patient. Figure 128 shows two different patients, one with a high fat (A) content and the other with a low fat (B) content.

Muscle Content

Patients who have excellent muscle tone and are very muscular pose a slightly more difficult problem in obtaining high quality images. The principal problem here is that the KvP should be increased due to the higher absorption rate of muscle. This adjustment compounds the radiographic contrast problem because, as was already mentioned, muscle produces large amounts of scatter by virtue of its high water content and increasing the KvP contributes additional quantities of scatter reaching the film. It has been the author's experience that it is very difficult to obtain a radiograph of high contrast in large, very muscular patients. In older patients, this muscle tissue will begin to slowly break down and will eventually become dehydrated to some extent, allowing considerably more x-rays to penetrate the body.

Water Content

Water content is a key indicator in detecting a healthy body, and too much or too little water has a deleterious effect on radiographic quality. Figure 125B shows a patient with excessive water in one side of the chest. Usually, it is unnecessary to penetrate the excess water; however, when it is necessary to do so, a more than moderate increase in KvP (approximately 15 to 30 depending on the initial KvP level and the quantity of water present) is usually indicated. Any additional increases to improve radiographic density should be made by increasing MaS and, as a last resort, a shorter focal film distance. The *proper content* of water in a healthy person helps to establish subject contrast of the body. With elderly patients, for example, dehydration and poor muscle tone require the technologist to reduce KvP, sometimes by as much as 10 to 20 in extreme cases, to help build subject contrast. As a result, the MaS should be increased to maintain proper radiographic density. Decreasing KvP under these conditions produces more differential absorption with less Compton interactions. At age 60, body water content is reduced to approximately 52 percent.

In general, radiography of older patients usually requires an overall reduction in exposure because of their poor absorption characteristics. The author's first rule of thumb is to reduce the KvP used to help increase subject contrast. In addition to this, a MaS reduction of 25 percent is often required for people between the ages of sixty-five and seventy-five, and for patients beyond eighty years of age a MaS reduction of 50 percent is often required.

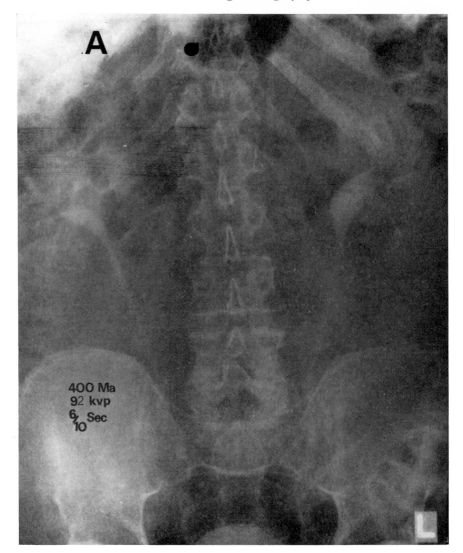

400 Ma
92 kvp
6/10 Sec

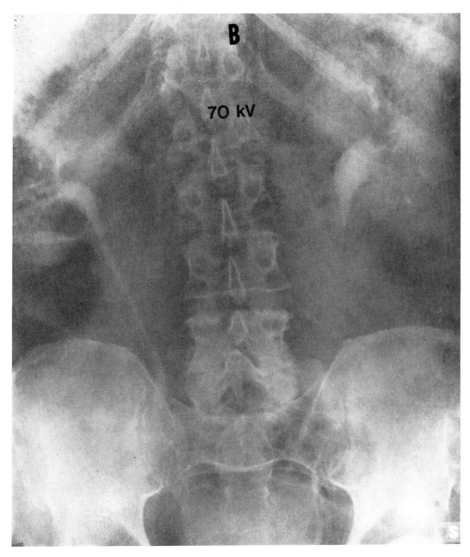

← Figure 127. Low KvP settings can improve subject contrast. Contrast is vastly improved in *B* as compared to *A*—the psoas muscles are more visible and the pelvic bone reveals considerably more detail. This was a large patient who measured 28 cm when lying supine.

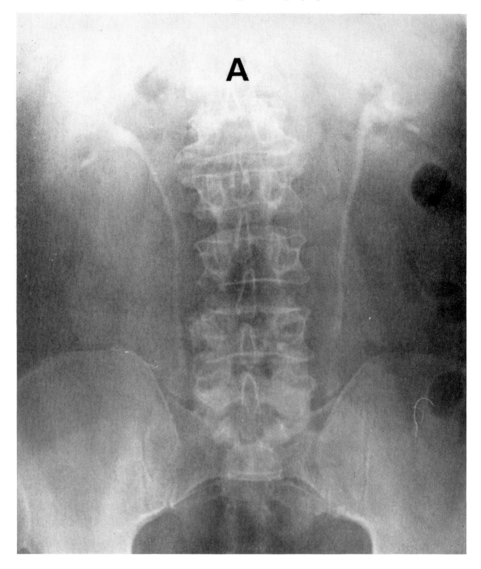

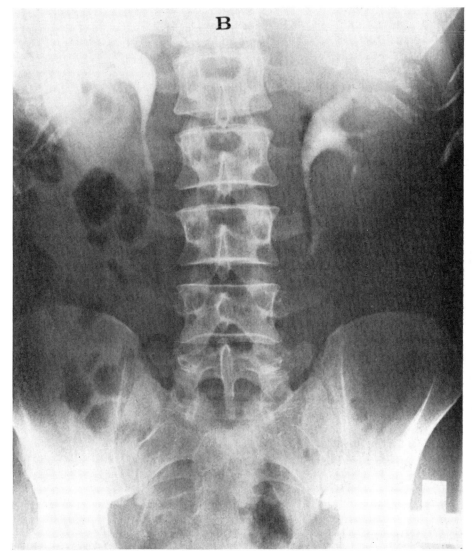

← Figure 128. Patients with different body compositions present vast differences for radiography. *A* was a middle-aged patient with a low subject contrast. *B* was a young patient with high subject contrast.

Bone Content

Bone content is the most consistent major body substance in terms of volume per patient (approximately 23 percent of body weight). It has a very low water content. It is interesting that bone has one of the most variable absorption qualities in radiography. The principle absorbing element in bone is calcium; the calcium content, however, changes widely with age. Figure 129 shows two radiographs demonstrating how the appearance of the bones of elderly people can be improved by reducing KvP. With elderly patients bony structures actually appear to be darker than the surrounding soft tissue.

Young children and infants also have low subject contrast between

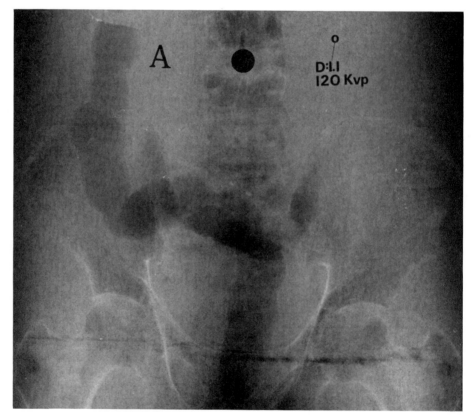

Figure 129A.

Figure 129. Greater differential absorptions can be achieved by reducing KvP and producing more photoelectric-type interactions; overall radiographic density has been maintained. Different KvP levels have been noted to demonstrate their effect when making such deliberate contrast adjustments. H & D curves are also shown. (A 12:1 grid was used throughout.)

bone and soft tissue. In either case, radiographic contrast between bone and soft tissue diminishes and makes diagnosis a very tricky proposition, especially when a fracture is small and the cortex remains in good alignment. The choice of technique for good bone radiography should be adjusted for age and possible pathology. As age increases, bone demineralizes and the beam's ability to penetrate quickly increases, thus producing an overall darker radiographic image. Due to this lack of absorption, it is felt by many that elderly patients should be exposed using a high MaS, low KvP type of technique. The diagnostic quality of the radiographs noted in Figure 129 is certainly an interesting comparison. The value of a less energetic beam with elderly patients becomes more understandable.

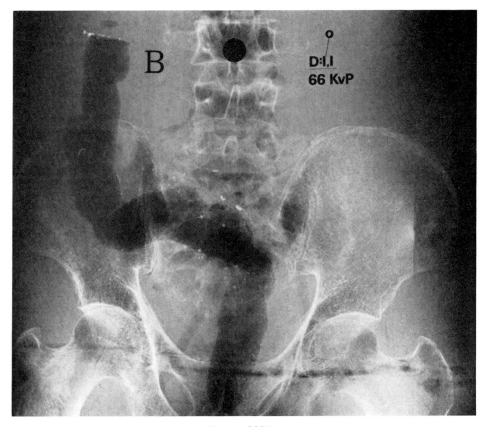

Figure 129B.

Pathology is another important item that contributes to a variation in bone absorption. A listing of common diseases that affect radiation absorption is shown in Figure 130.

From the above discussion, the technologist should keep in mind that

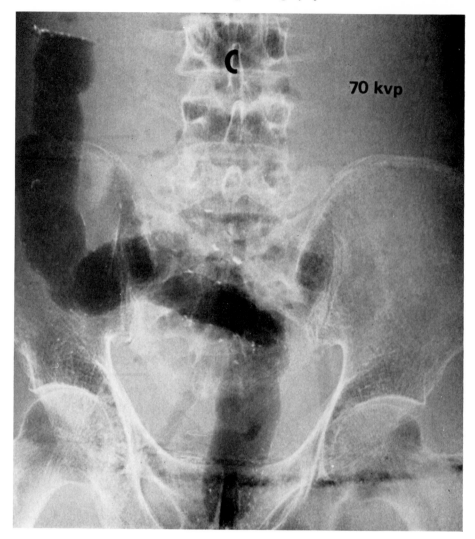

Figure 129C.

the mention of a specific disease in the patient's history might well be noted because possible adjustments in technique may be necessary.

Evaluating the Patient

It is important for the technologist to be able to "size up" the patient correctly before the first exposure is made. During the first few minutes with the patient as much attention as possible should be paid to such things as overall muscle tone, age, fat, muscle content, and possible pathology, and in reviewing the patient's history. While helping the patient on the table, one might be noting how firm the muscular structure is and

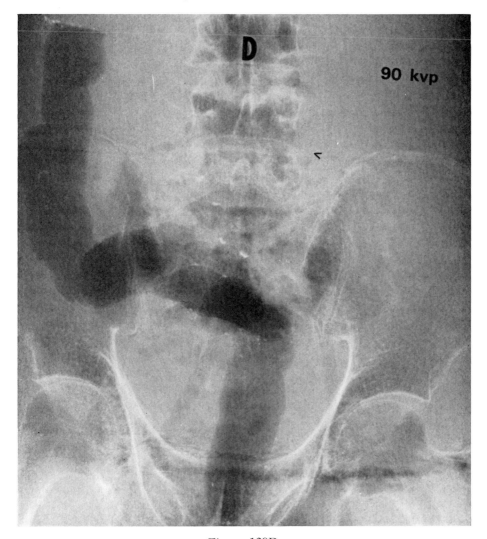

Figure 129D.

the overall mass of the patient. Considering these aspects along with age and pathology, the technologist is better able to have the body habitus "pigeonholed" or "sized up" pretty well. Remember that no one factor thus far mentioned is sufficient, singularly, as a determining factor for establishing a technique. Through experience and careful observation, a competent technologist develops an intuitive awareness as to how the primary beam will be modified by the patient's body. In Chapters Eleven and Twelve suggestions will be presented regarding how one can juggle exposure factors to arrive at a technique that would be most likely to produce an optimal radiographic image. The manner with which adjusting exposure factors is accomplished, from the author's point of view, makes the differentiation between a "button pusher" and a skilled professional radiographic technologist.

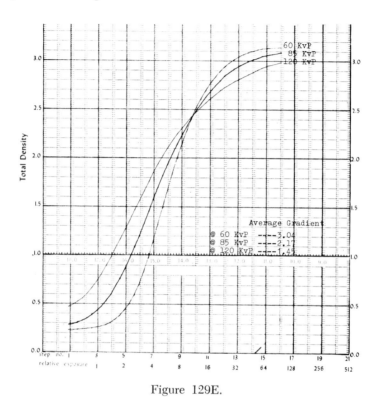

Figure 129E.

Figure 130. Common diseases that often affect the radiographic image. The technologist should refer to the patient's history for clues in determining the final exposure factors.

COMMON PATHOLOGICAL FACTORS

Increased Tissue Density

Condition	Commonly Seen In
Osteoblastic Metastases	Bones
Paget's Disease	Bones
Pleural Effusion (Accumulation Of Fluid)	Chest
Consolidated Lungs (Pneumonia)	Chest
Intra-abdominal Fluid (Ascites)	Abdomen

Decreased Tissue Density

Condition	Commonly Seen In
Osteoporosis	Bones
Emphysema	Chest
Bowel Obstruction (Excessive Abdominal Air)	Abdomen

IMPORTANT CHARACTERISTICS OF MAJOR BODY REGIONS

The body can be separated into four major regions: (1) the abdomen, (2) the chest, (3) the extremities, and (4) the skull. Each of these requires the use of a different combination of exposure factors. A brief discussion of the differences and similarities of these regions will prove beneficial in understanding how various body regions influence the overall radiographic image. Also, some insight might be gained regarding the different philosophies held by various radiologists and technologists as to which set of exposure factors may produce the best results.

The Chest Region

Earlier, the concept of subject contrast was presented. To review quickly, subject contrast is a comparison of the rates at which various body structures absorb the primary beam. If an area is constructed in such a way that it produces obvious or abrupt differences in absorption rates, it is said to have high subject contrast. If, on the other hand, the inherent absorption ability of the various body tissues in the region under examination are similar, we identify it as having a low subject contrast which would produce low radiographic contrast.

The chest region has a relatively high subject contrast. A brief analysis of its components will explain why. First, there is normally a considerable amount of air in the chest, and air is commonly considered an effective contrast media. In a manner of speaking, most of the structures in the chest are bathed in or surrounded by air, which causes great variations in absorption rate. The effect of this is shown in Figure 131. You can see the object under examination is less obvious in "A" than it is in "B" with the presence of air being the only variable. Second, the structures of the chest are not as compact as those of the abdomen and thus are generally easier to distinguish. The third major factor that contributes to high subject contrast is the density of the structures present in the chest. For example, the structures of the mediastinum are extremely dense when compared to lung tissue. The major vessels contain fluid and so they are much more absorbent to x-rays than the air filled lungs that surround them. In short, wide variations between tissue density, a moderate degree of separation between structures, the presence of large amounts of air and, of course, the various mixture of major body tissues all contribute to the high subject contrast of the chest region.

The Abdomen

The abdomen presents an altogether different problem to the technologist. Here, the structures and organs involved have a much more

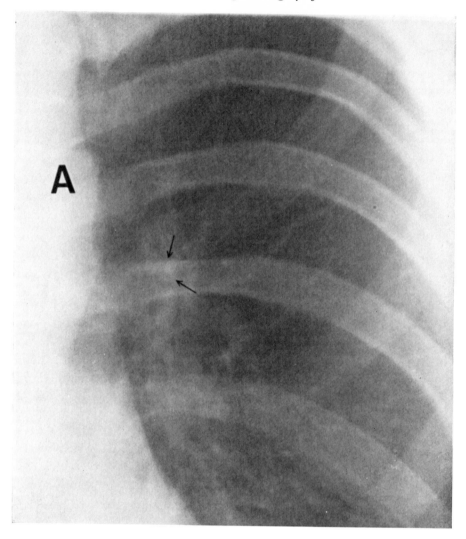

subtle subject contrast; thus, the abdominal area is known to have a rather *low subject* contrast. The relative water content of the abdomen area is high, and tissue density of the structures in the abdomen are very uniform as compared to those of the chest. Another important factor is that the various organs in the abdomen have similar absorption characteristics and are often partly superimposed on each other. This, of course, makes it even more difficult for the beam to distinguish between the absorption rate of one tissue as opposed to that of another. The end result is a remnant beam that is very uniform as it reaches the film. The presence of fat, however, tends to silhouette some organs in the radiographic image providing a slight increase in the visibility of the structures. In fact, the

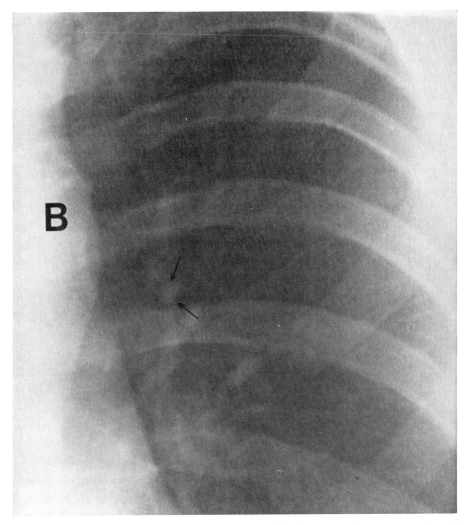

← Figure 131. The small node (arrow) in A is difficult to see when compared to the same node in B, shifted to a slightly different location by respiration.

absence of these fatty layers around various organs is sometimes indicative of disease. The kidney is a good example of this, as noted in Figure 132. Also, the thickness of each organ plays an important role in the ultimate subject contrast, and of course the absence of air makes the overall absorption rates even more uniform.

The Extremities

The extremities have the greatest subject contrast in its strictest sense. Each extremity has only two major tissues that absorb the x-ray beam:

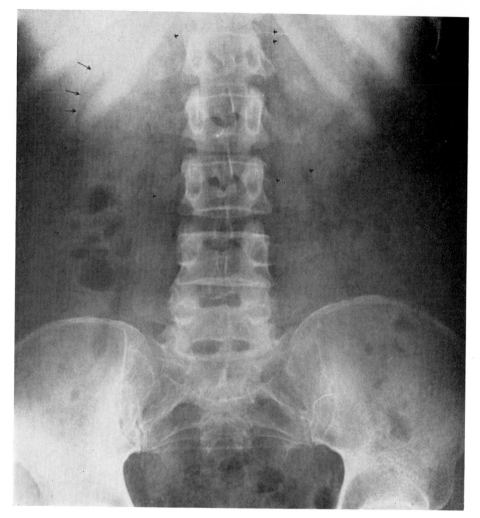

Figure 132. A number of "fatty" lines are indicated, others are not indicated.

the bone and the surrounding muscle. Thus, with extremities the two major absorption rates are bone versus soft tissue. With this arrangement of subject contrast, the differences in absorption rates are great.

The Skull

The skull offers a problem still different from those already discussed. The skull, of course, involves pure bone radiography. There is very little soft tissue to diagnose or reproduce radiographically, so the subject contrast of this area is primarily caused by various thicknesses of the bone. The petrous bone offers a definite change in absorption relative to the external wall of the skull. The areas of the face have some cavities in which air can commonly be seen. As you already know, varying thickness of any similar tissue including soft tissue can affect subject contrast.

A LOOK AT PHOTON-TISSUE INTERACTIONS

It should be kept clearly in mind that no diagnostic exposure possesses only a single type of interaction, but rather a mixture of interactions. There is, however, a dominant type of interaction for each exposure and that interaction is largely responsible for the resultant radiographic effect (see Fig. 133).

In Chapter Seven much time was given to describe how the various types of interactions affect radiographic contrast as controlled by the KvP level. We should now approach this topic with slightly more detail so the technologist's scope of understanding will be appropriately widened. Before going on, we should recall the three possible situations the primary beam may experience: complete penetration of the body parts, an interaction involving partial absorption produced by the Compton effect, and the interaction involving total absorption caused by photoelectric interactions. There are other interactions that can occur in the body as a result of irradiation; however, for the kilovoltages used in diagnostic radiography, the Compton and photoelectric interactions are primarily responsible for producing the radiographic image, and our discussion will be limited to these.

It should be very apparent by now that the interaction between body tissues and the beam of x-ray photons is the central issue in radiography. It has been the author's opinion for some time that, whether radiography is viewed primarily as a science or as an art, technologists must have a clear understanding as to how x-rays interact with body tissues to produce the remnant beam, because it is, after all, the remnant beam that will ultimately determine radiographic quality. The scope of this discussion on x-ray interactions with tissue will be brief and oriented to its very practical applications.

Photoelectric Interaction

The photoelectric interaction is interesting and very important to radiography. It involves the production of two types of secondary radiation, while the original primary photon disappears altogether. It should be pointed out and kept in mind throughout this discussion that the KvP level used for any exposure primarily determines the type of interaction that eventually results. The photoelectric effect, for example, is more likely to occur in the 35 to 70 KvP range.

A schematic of the photoelectric interaction can be seen in Figure 134. The incident photon strikes an electron located in one of the inner orbits;

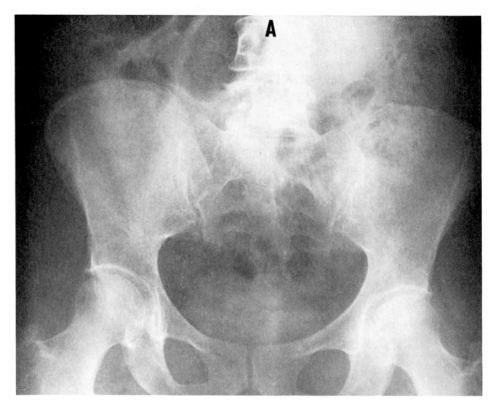

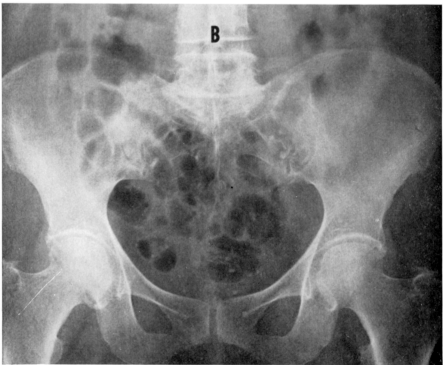

Figure 133. The KvP is increased in *A* as compared to *B*. The resulting increase in Compton interactions in *A* produced a more homogenic density pattern on the film. (These patients had a very similar body habitus.)

usually only the K or L shells are involved. The first thing that becomes apparent is that the entering photon disappears entirely. It is totally absorbed by the atom of the tissue, which now suddenly has more energy than it knows what to do with. By referring to the law of conservation of energy, we know that a form of energy (such as an x-ray photon) cannot simply disappear without any other effect. Immediately, the excited atom ejects an electron from one of its innermost shells in an attempt to balance its overall energy state. The ejected electron is called, as it begins its voyage from its home shell, a photoelectron. The photoelectron has less energy than the original primary x-ray photon that struck the atom. By further inspection of Figure 134, you will see that an electron from an

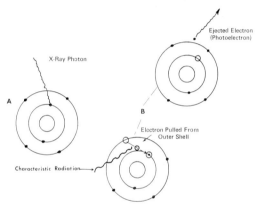

PHOTOELECTRIC INTERACTION

Figure 134. An entering primary x-ray photon strikes the L shell and is totally consumed. The atom cannot contain this increased energy and discards it by ejecting an electron. The emitted photoelectron will probably not go through more than a few centimeters of body tissue before being absorbed. An electron is moved inward to fill the vacancy; because it is going to an orbit with a lower energy level, it discards its excess energy, known as characteristic radiation. The characteristic radiation travels an even shorter distance in the body before it is absorbed. The photoelectric effect is thus a total absorption interaction.

outer shell moves to fill the vacancy in the inner orbital shell, but to be "comfortable" in its new location, it must adjust its own energy to the energy level of its new home. This is accomplished by emitting what is known as characteristic radiation. The term *characteristic* is used here because it tells something about the element or orbit from which the radiation came. There is a cascading series of new electrons that serves to satisfy the other orbital vacancies, and each produces its appropriate level of characteristic radiation. This process will continue until all vacancies of the atom are filled and the atom is once again stable. The outer

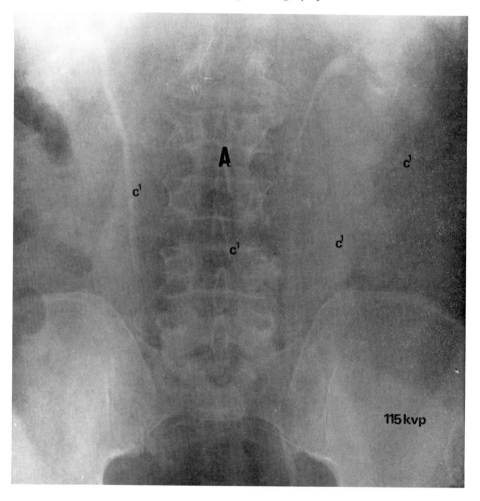

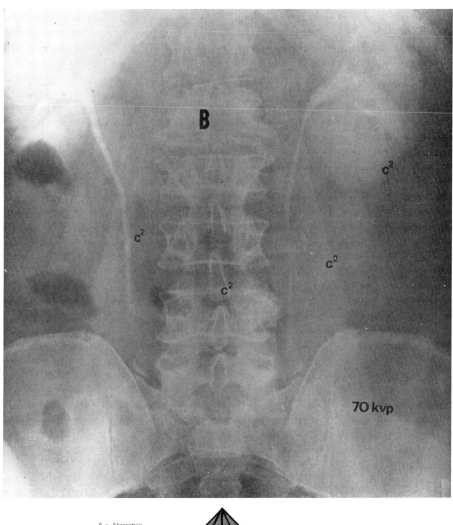

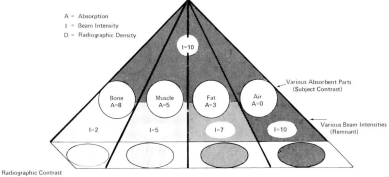

A = Absorption
I = Beam Intensity
D = Radiographic Density

Various Absorbent Parts
(Subject Contrast)

I=10

Bone
A=8

Muscle
A=5

Fat
A=3

Air
A=0

I=2

I=5

I=7

I=10

Various Beam Intensities
(Remnant)

Radiographic Contrast

← Figure 135. Differences in body part absorptions are always present to some extent in a diagnostic exposure. The degree of difference is dependent on the type of interaction, which is determined by the beam's energy level. The "C" numbers tell the variance between the radiographic densities in adjacent body structures. This comparison indicates that a higher radiographic contrast is achieved when a lower KvP is used because it increases differential absorption.

shell will fill its vacancy by pulling in a free floating electron which may be moving in the general vicinity of the vacancy.

The importance of this interaction to the radiographic image is that it is extremely sensitive to tissues having different atomic numbers and absorption rates. This means that with a particular exposure, body tissues having different atomic numbers, i.e. fat, bone, muscle, and air, and different tissue densities would have corresponding absorption differences. These differences in body absorption will cause corresponding differences in the intensities of remnant radiation which will, in turn, expose the film to varying degrees. Figure 135 shows this concept schematically. It should be kept in mind that it was the kilovoltage level that made the photo-electric effect dominant in this particular exposure. If another kilovoltage was chosen (above 70 KvP) a different type of interaction would more likely result and the effect of this would be the production of a radiographic image with a different overall appearance.

The photoelectric interaction can be used by the technologist to gain relatively high subject contrast. There are certain examinations that demand high absorption variations (subject contrast) in the body. With IVP examinations, for example, it is important that not only the kidney be seen easily but the opacified calyces be optimally visible as well. There is obviously a difference in atomic number between the kidney and the contrast material and, by using the photoelectric effect, one can take advantage of this and produce the best technical image possible. Most iodine-based contrast material gives optimal opacification when irradiated by Kv levels from 60 to 70. Figure 135 shows two radiographs using high and low KvP levels. While reviewing these radiographs, it should be brought to mind that the type of interaction that was dominant during these exposures has a great influence on the contrast of the radiographic image and that the type of interaction can be effectively controlled by the choice of kilovoltage.

One last example might be helpful to cement this concept in the reader's mind. Rib examinations are often difficult to radiograph; in fact, it is the author's opinion that they are one of the most technically difficult studies of all. There is, however, an extreme difference in the atomic numbers of the internal thoracic structures and the bony thorax. If one keeps this in mind and uses the principles described above regarding the photoelectric effect and low KvP, one has a considerably better chance of producing a good diagnostic study. One should not let the physical size of the patient intimidate one's thinking. For a chest measuring 28 cm A.P., a surprisingly low KvP (50 to 60) is adequate for penetration. At these Kv levels, the photoelectric interaction will go to work on the technologist's behalf, taking advantage of the relatively large differences in atomic number between the lungs, bone, air, and vessels to produce optimal contrast. Of course, for chest radiography, high KvP exposures would more likely produce optimal radiographs.

Compton Interaction (Modified Scattering)

The Compton interaction or Compton effect is shown in Figure 136, where an incident photon is striking a loosely bound outer electron. The angle at which the primary photon makes "contact" with the outer orbiting electron will determine how much energy the photon loses and what direction it will take afterward. If a high energy photon strikes the outer electron at a glancing (indirect) angle, it will lose less of its original photon energy to the atom than if it were traveling on a more direct course. An analogy of how billiard balls react when they strike each other at different angles and with varying speeds can be useful here. The incident primary photon, upon contact with the orbiting electron, leaves the interaction site with a different angle as a cue ball would. The primary photon after this collision with the electron is known as a scattered photon. During this interaction the outer electron will be dislodged from its orbit and is then called a recoil or Compton electron. The vacancy is filled by a free, floating electron. There is some characteristic radiation given off as the vacancy is filled by the free electron, but it is so low in energy it has no effect on the radiographic image as with the photoelectron.

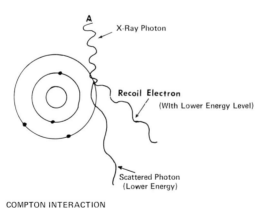

COMPTON INTERACTION

Figure 136. As a result of the collision of a higher energy primary x-ray photon with another orbiting electron, a recoil electron (called a Compton electron) is ejected from the atom. Simultaneously, a scattered photon is produced and exposes the film.

In general, as the KvP is increased, the role of the Compton interaction in producing the ultimate radiographic image is increased. There are two reasons for this. First, as the KvP is increased, the relative number of

Compton interactions as compared to photoelectric interactions increases. Second, with increased KvP the scattered photons are more penetrating *and* are directed more toward the film. The increased penetrability of the scattered radiation compiled with a greater tendency to travel toward the film results in a definite increase in radiographic fog. The methods used to control radiographic fog produced by excessive scatter will be discussed thoroughly in Chapter Nine. Figure 137 shows how scatter photons cause this unnecessary and unwanted radiographic density known as fog. After rambling around inside the patient, the *scattered* photons are either absorbed by the patient or go on to expose the film. Overall, considerably more of these photons expose the film as opposed to those that are absorbed by the body. Those that strike the film do so with indifference to the body's inherent subject contrast. In other words, the scattered photons are likely to expose an area of the film that is supposed to be light in density. The net effect of this is that crucial differences in radiographic densities are greatly diminished, and the diagnostic value of the image is seriously impaired.

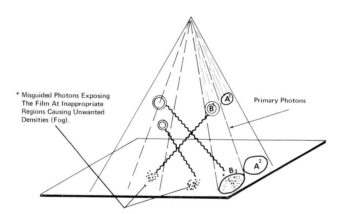

Figure 137. Object A has totally absorbed the primary x-ray and is recorded by the film with a light density. Object B produces a scatter photon as a result of partial primary beam absorption; scatter photons have invaded the area of the film noted as B², causing that area to be fogged. In reality, this invasion of scatter photons is evenly spread across the entire film, producing an overall gray flat radiographic image.

Between the photoelectric and Compton interaction, the probability of a photon emitted by the x-ray tube passing through the patient without undergoing some type of interaction is relatively low. It has been estimated that less than 10 percent of the beam reaches the film in its original form. With this fact, one can see more easily how important these interactions are in radiography.

Summary

In all, the body causes the final adjustment or modification of the x-ray beam before it reaches the film. Differences in absorption (subject contrast) among various body tissue types will determine, to a great extent, the ultimate radiographic quality. When one considers that up to 90 percent of the radiation exiting the patient is not directly produced by the target (not primary radiation) of the x-ray tube, but rather by the body itself, we can more realistically appreciate the body as an emitter of x-rays: This knowledge demands our strict attention as technologists.

In general the patient must be evaluated in total. A patient's age or weight simply does not supply one with enough important information about the patient's absorbing characteristics. Similarly, measurements alone should not be used as a single source of data for establishing a set of exposure factors. The patient's abdomen which measures 21 cm A.P. actually tells you very little. The patient could be 90 years old; he could be athletic with excellent muscle tone; or he could be a middle-aged individual with a large degree of fat content. Each one of these conditions should signal the technologist that an adjustment might be necessary beyond the technique chart. In short, there is no real substitute for experience in making the final judgment in technique. One should be mindful, however, that mere seniority is not an accurate measure of experience. There are unfortunately a number of technologists who have been working for a number of years, but due to a lack of professional interest and self-discipline in relating theory to practical application, their "real" experience is quite limited.

FILTRATION AND RADIOGRAPHY

There is one remaining factor that must be discussed. Although important, from a practical point of view, it is a factor over which the technologist has little or no control. All *routine* diagnostic exposures are made with a filter fixed between the x-ray tube and the collimator. A filter is used to reduce the number of unnecessary photons reaching the body. The main concern here is obviously one of radiation safety and patient dose. It is well known that many low energy x-rays are emitted by the tube during each diagnostic exposure. Their effect radiographically is of no significance; however, they do produce unnecessary photon interactions (ionizations) in the body which, of course, increase the patient's dose. To prevent this, a thin aluminum filter is placed between the portal of the x-ray tube and the collimator aperature. There is always some inherent filtration provided by the glass envelope and surrounding oil which is usually equal to from 0.5 to 1.0 mm aluminum. To this, equipment manufacturers generally add at least 2.0 mm Al of "additional filtration." The inherent filtration (in the glass envelope) plus the added filtration produces a total filtration equal to no less than 2.5 mm to meet government regulations. When low KvP values are required, perhaps for special soft tissue techniques, less total filtration can be used since government standards for filtration are calculated according to the "probable" KvP level that is most likely to be used by the equipment.

The Radiographic Effect of Filtration

One can easily see by viewing Figure 138 that only moderate radiographic differences are produced as a result of commonly used filter thicknesses, as long as one does not exceed 3.0 mm aluminum. Filtration produces a harder beam because the filter absorbs the many soft rays that would cause the overall primary beam to be softer. As filtration increases to a certain point beyond normal diagnostic thicknesses, the overall beam becomes excessively harder. The effect of adding filtration to the beam has some similarities to increasing the KvP.

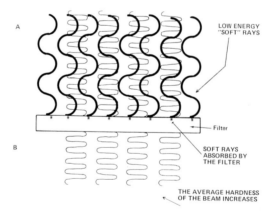

Figure 138. As filtration thickness increases, fewer and fewer x-rays can penetrate, resulting in decreased radiographic density. Fewer lower energy photons pass through the filter as thickness increases, and higher energy photons reach the film. The average energy of the beam is higher and more uniform.

The radiographic effect caused by filters is that of decreased contrast and decreased density. It was pointed out earlier that the objective of filtration is to remove lower energy, diagnostically useless x-rays. With light filtration this is true; however, as thicker filters (greater than 3.0) are used, there is some absorption of the higher energy rays. Contrast is decreased with increasing filtration thicknesses because the beam's penetrating capability is more uniform (as shown in Fig. 139). This will cause

a more even penetration of the various body parts giving rise to less subject contrast. In short, the advantage of filtration is basically to prevent
unnecessary exposure to the patient by absorbing those soft rays that have
no radiographic effect. It should be noted from a radiation safety point
of view that, if a technologist notices or even suspects that a filter is not
being used properly, he should report his suspicions to his supervisor without delay. Further, one should not attempt to repair or make any adjustments in filtration, but leave this specialized work to a trained service
person.

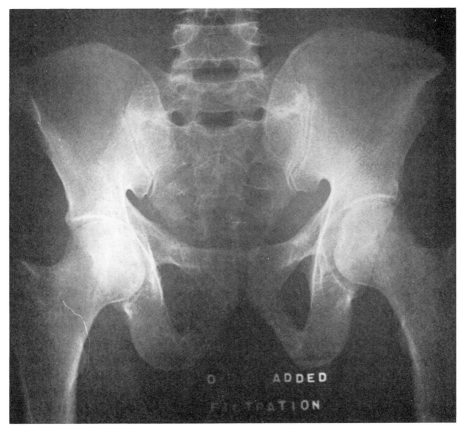

Figure 139A.

Figure 139. As filtration increases, density and contrast decrease.

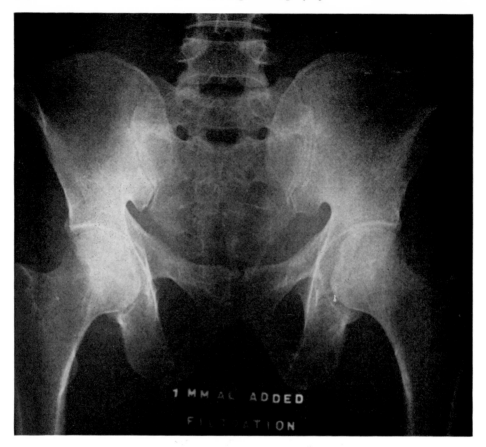

Figure 139B.

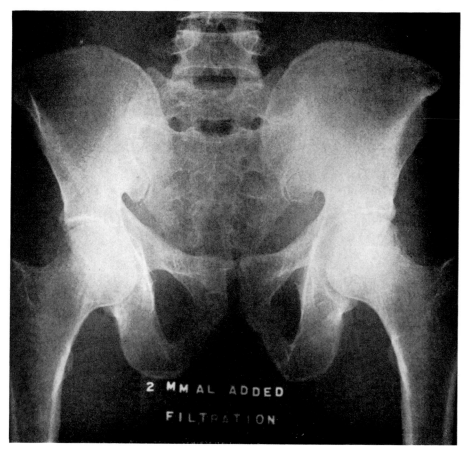

Figure 139C.

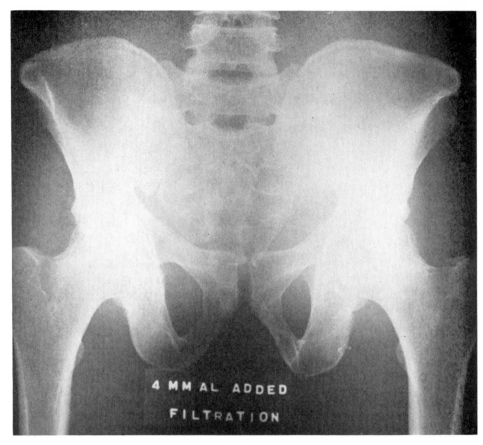

Figure 139D.

CHAPTER NINE

CONTROLLING THE REMNANT BEAM

R ECOGNIZING THE INFLUENCE the remnant beam has on the radiographic image, this chapter will discuss the accessory equipment used by the technologist to control its effects on the image. Primarily, scatter radiation will be of major concern here.

THE CONCEPT OF CONING

We have established thus far that the presence of *excess* scatter radiation in a remnant beam will produce a fogged image. It should be emphasized here that excessive scatter radiation is determined by the ratio of primary photons to scatter photons making up the remnant beam. One way for the technologist to control this unwanted proportion of scatter radiation is to limit the numbers of interactions that produce scatter within the patient.

Reducing the number of interactions within the patient at first sounds like a complicated process. The use of coning, however, is extremely helpful in this regard and can be used without difficulty. Coning or beam-limiting devices control the amount of S/S interactions by simply restricting field size. Researchers realize that because S/S rays travel toward the film in such varying directions it seems reasonable to presume a scattered photon could be produced in one area of the body and strike an entirely different area of the film's emulsion. Figure 140 shows this effect. It can be understood that when a technologist is doing an examination of the gallbladder, for example, S/S radiation could strike an area of the film located in a region of the lumbar spine, kidney, or pelvis. These "transplanted" rays can be easily controlled with the use of beam limiting devices and with the use of radiographic grids. We have seen how S/S radiation can indeed stray from the point of origin to another location on the film surface. This causes what would normally be light areas of the film to have an additional density and decreased radiographic contrast results. The major contributor to radiographic fog is an excess amount of scatter rays in the remnant beam.

Types of Beam-Limiting Devices

There are four types of beam-limiting or restricting devices: (1) general purpose cones; (2) cylinder cones; (3) diaphragms; and (4) collima-

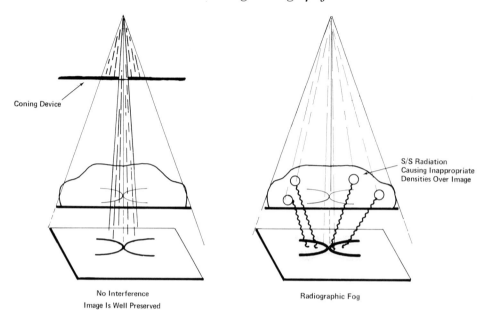

Coning Device

S/S Radiation
Causing Inappropriate
Densities Over Image

No Interference
Image Is Well Preserved

Radiographic Fog

Figure 140. Unwanted densities are produced by scattered photons causing a general decrease in contrast of the object under examination.

tors (see Fig. 141). Collimators have become the most important of these because of the advantages they offer in patient safety and in convenience to the technologist. Also, government legislation aimed at reducing the patient exposure to unnecessary radiation has encouraged the use of collimators. This legislation prescribes that all newly purchased collimators must be electrically connected to the bucky tray so that it will automatically cone down to the film size used. The technologist now has considerably fewer options over coning as compared to recent years. Until about 1960, mostly cylinder and general purpose type cones were used. Because they were not adjustable, hurried technologists often did not change cone sizes with each size of film used. As a result, cones were not always properly used and the patient did occasionally receive additional unnecessary doses, while films had decreased radiographic quality. Manufacturers were urged to produce a device that would be less time-consuming for technologists to use and would provide better radiation protection for patients; modern collimators provide the answer. With this device, quick adjustments in field size can be easily accomplished.

Basic Construction of a Collimator

Collimators, regardless of the manufacturer, have basically the same components, which include a light source used for centering the central ray over the body part, a mirror to project the light beam to the patient, and a series of pulleys to move a pair of lead plates. The important value of having a light source is to show the technologist what area of the body will be irradiated so that proper positioning can more easily be accomplished.

The mirror must be held firmly in a precise position inside the collimator or the projected light coming out of the collimator will not give a true guide for centering (as noted in Fig. 141). Complaints that centering locks on the tube crane have gone out of adjustment or that the table is off center often reveal that the mirror had slipped out of adjustment and that the locks themselves and the table are in good working order.

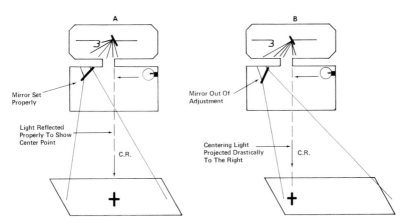

Figure 141. The mirror is responsible for projecting the collimator's light properly. The repair work should be done by a service person, not a technologist.

A well-designed collimator will have built into it a double set of adjustable lead leafs. A double pair as opposed to a single pair of lead leafs provides increased coning at the edges.

Besides the mirror slipping out of adjustment, another problem that will occur with collimators is that the shutters themselves could go out of adjustment. This is often a result of small cables slipping and getting caught in the nylon pulleys. It should be clearly understood that any corrections involving a beam-limiting device should be left strictly to a trained service person because any adjustments in field size or alignment possess a potential radiation safety hazard to the patient and to the technologist.

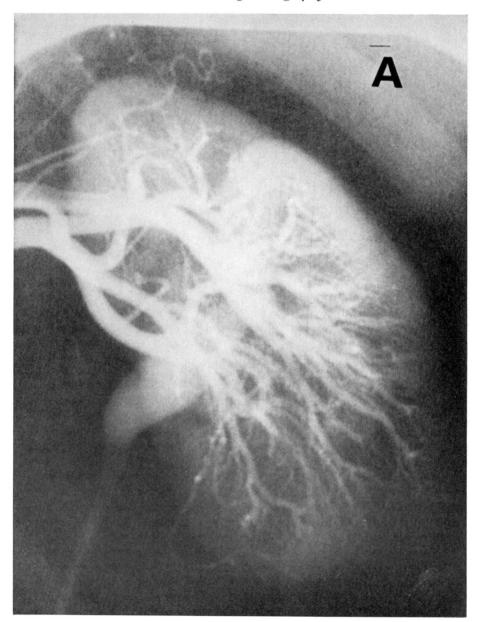

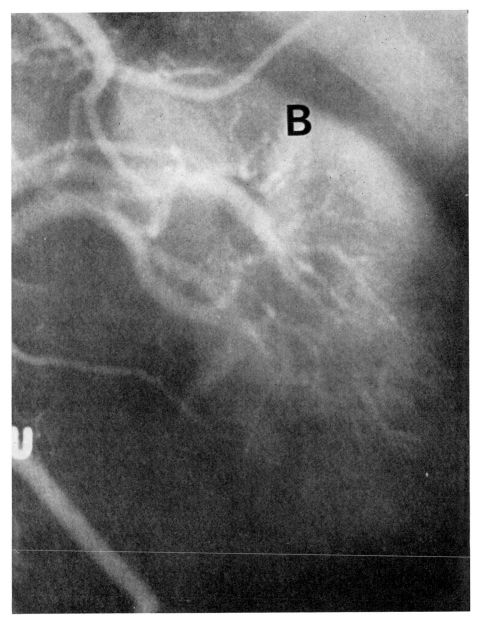

← Figure 142. Very "tight" coning in this examination has a positive effect. Increased contrast has improved visibility of detail greatly in *A*.

Uses for Conventional Cones

Of the conventional type cones that have been used before the collimator, cylinders are still favored for many special radiographic procedures such as tightly coned down selective renal arteriograms or cerebral arteriograms. Figure 142 shows a selective renal arteriogram using a cylinder cone and is compared to an open field exposure.

THE RADIOGRAPHIC EFFECT OF BEAM-LIMITING DEVICES

The purpose of using a beam-limiting device is to reduce unnecessary exposure to the patient and to improve radiographic contrast by reducing the number of scatter interactions in the patient. With this, since S/S rays are photons with penetrating qualities that help produce radiographic density, the technologist should be mindful that when their numbers are reduced radiographic density is moderately to significantly decreased. In

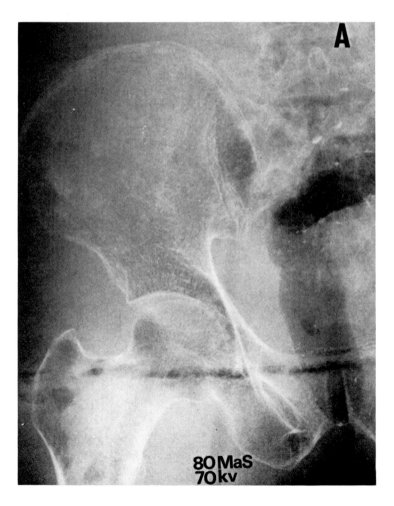

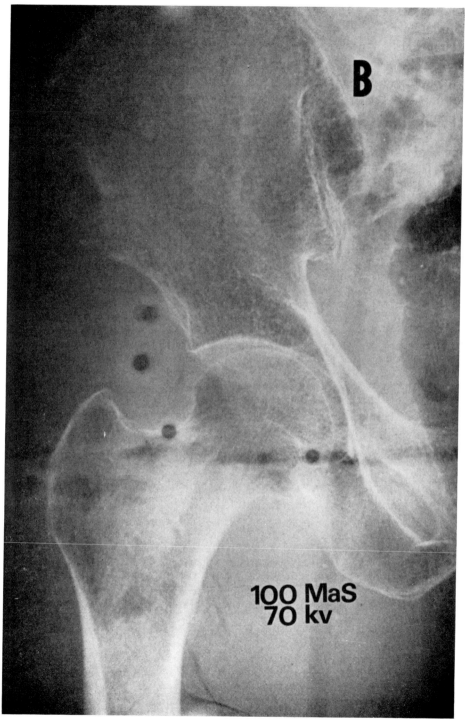

← Figure 143. The MaS has been increased by 25 percent to compensate for coning.

addition to the density issue, increased coning causes a moderate to substantial increase in radiographic contrast as well. It is generally understood that when moderately tighter coning is used where it was not previously at least a 5 Kv increase is necessary to regain the lost density. From the author's point of view, however, it would be more appropriate to increase the MaS by 25 percent to 35 percent (depending on the total amount of S/S produced). Reasons for this are, first, increments of 5 KvP do not always produce the same radiographic effect at all Kv levels because of the Kv influence on exposure latitude, and, second, increasing KvP is likely to produce more scatter interactions which will tend to defeat the purpose of the coning. The effect on the radiographic image is determined by the thickness of the body part, to what extent coning has been used, the level of KvP being used, the density of the body, and the atomic number (type of tissue) being irradiated. In Figure 143 we can see the degree of compensation used when tight coning was employed as compared to open field.

Influences on Patient Dose

As was pointed out earlier, field size has a strong influence on the total number of interactions within the patient. In reality, it is the interaction that accounts for the danger in irradiating patients. At normal settings, an A-P lumbar spine exam exposed with and without coning will result in differing exposure doses to the patient. To say the least, the technologist must be especially mindful of coning procedures when radiographing children and young adults of child-bearing years.

Summary

The important concept for the technologist to remember regarding beam limiting is that excess amounts of S/S radiation (disproportionate quantities of secondary to primary) are strongly influenced by exposing too large an area of the patient's body part. The resulting overabundance of scatter rays causes high volumes of radiographic fog which in turn produces poor radiographic contrast. With the use of beam limiting devices, smaller field sizes can be obtained, causing fewer numbers of interactions to form (less stray or transplanted rays). This sequence of events usually improves contrast and visibility of detail.

⋀ Field size leads to ⋀ S/S interaction resulting in S/S rays striking the film producing ⋀ Density and ⋁ Contrast.

Although contrast improves with progressively tighter coning, the most dramatic radiographic effect occurs when going from no coning to a cone of the correct size for the body part under examination and when the smallest cone cylinders are used for spot filming. It should not be forgotten that different body parts produce varying quantities of scatter, and that proper coning is very important for those areas that yield large quantities of scatter. With this in mind, it should be clear that when adjusting the technique for coning situations, one should be mindful of the total amount of scatter radiation produced by that particular body part. For example, tight coning will have much less effect on density and contrast when radiographing an elbow than it would if the same coning changes were made when radiographing an abdomen or a lateral lumbar spine.

RADIOGRAPHIC GRIDS

The Concept

Although coning is effective in improving radiographic contrast by reducing field size, it must be kept in mind that, even if proper coning is used, the body part under examination provides sufficient quantities of S/S radiation to cause S/S fog. Thus, a device must be placed in the remnant beam that will further reduce the amount of S/S rays.

You have already learned how adjustments in KvP will alter the number and type of interactions produced by a body part, but this alone does not sufficiently improve radiographic quality and, in addition, increases the possibility of underpenetration.

The grid is actually a kind of "filter" that absorbs radiation attempting to pass through its lead strips *at too great a divergent angle* as compared with the primary beam. Figure 144 shows that, with all the negative characteristics associated with scatter radiation, it is fortunate that they travel

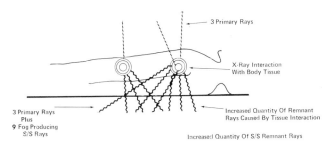

Figure 144. Many more scatter photons than primary photons reach the film. Scatter photons travel in very different patterns as compared to primary photons, especially when lower KvP exposures are used. The numbers used do not indicate actual values.

at a more divergent angle than the primary photons. In fact, this one characteristic of S/S makes the use of grids practical. The total S/S filtering effect, known as *cleanup*, is mainly regulated by grid ratio. Grid ratio is the relationship between the height of the lead strip to the distance between them.

Construction

Radiographic grids are available in a number of types and styles, yet all grids are composed of nothing more than a series of alternating lead strips (cut very thin) and radiolucent material. The type of radiolucent substance most used for this interspace material is aluminum, although in some cases, especially in the older grids, cardboard is used. Cardboard interspacing is not as popular now because it is not as strong as the other material and also has some sensitivity to humidity changes causing expansion and contraction. With this expansion and contraction over time, the very thin lead strips become warped and cause radiographic defects.

Aluminum interspacing material, as might be expected, has a slight advantage because it usually has a somewhat higher absorption rate to scatter rays, resulting in slightly better cleanup.

Grid Ratio

One of the most important characteristics manufactured into a grid is its ratio. Grid ratio, by definition, is the relationship between the height of the lead strip and the spaces between. Common grid ratios are 5:1, 6:1, 8:1, 10:1, 12:1. The use of 16:1 grids has very little advantage in cleanup and relatively high disadvantage in narrow positioning latitude which will be discussed later; as a result, 16:1 grids are becoming less popular. A 5:1 grid, for example, will contain lead strips measuring five times higher than the actual distance between them (see Fig. 145). Grid

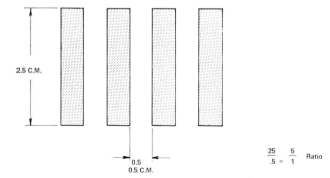

Figure 145. The relationship between the height of the lead and the interspace will greatly affect the likelihood of the grid trapping more or fewer scatter photons.

ratio principally determines what percent of scatter it can remove from the remnant beam. The percentage of scatter removed from the beam as earlier noted is called cleanup or grid efficiency. As more scatter rays are taken out of the remnant beam by the grid, the grid is said to have better cleanup and greater efficiency.

Although it will be no surprise to hear that cleanup increases as grid ratio increases, it is important to know that the increase in cleanup is *not* proportionate with increases in grid ratio. For example, the cleanup for a 5:1 grid is approximately 88 percent (removes 88% of S/S in the remnant beam); but if a 10:1 grid ratio is used in place of a 5:1, the cleanup will be approximately 91.2 percent, which represents an additional cleanup of only approximately 4 percent. As still higher grid ratios are used, additional cleanup becomes even less dramatic. When going from a 12:1 grid to a 16:1 grid, the additional cleanup in S/S is only 3 percent and the effect on the radiographic image is very slight, indeed. The radiographic effect of using a grid is more obvious when higher KvPs are used with thick, dense body parts (see Fig. 146). In general terms, it can be correctly stated that as grid ratio increases grid efficiency and cleanup increase as well. Figure 147 shows the relative increases in cleanup using various grid ratios. There is, of course, a decrease in density because (1) less S/S is reaching the film and (2) grids do absorb some primary photons.

| GRID RATIO | 60 KvP | | 100 KvP | |
	% OF SCATTER ABSORPTION	% OF PRIMARY ABSORPTION	% OF SCATTER ABSORPTION	% OF PRIMARY ABSORPTION
5:1	88%	approx 30%	70%	24.2%
6:1	89.4%	– – –	81%	– – – –
8:1	93%	31.4%	88.8%	27%
12:1	95.8%	34.3%	92.5%	29.1%
16:1	97.2%	35.6%	95.4%	31.6%
5:1 cross	97.6%	53.8%	92.6%	39%
8:1 cross	99.1%	50 8%	97%	46.3%

Figure 146.

In quick review, as grid ratio increases more S/S radiation is removed from the remnant beam thereby providing a better balance of scatter to primary in the remnant beam; less S/S radiation reaches the film, and the radiographic image will have slightly greater contrast thus providing the technologist and radiologist with much better visibility of detail. Because the amount of cleanup is mainly determined by ratio, progressively higher grid ratios will progressively produce higher radiographic contrasts. In

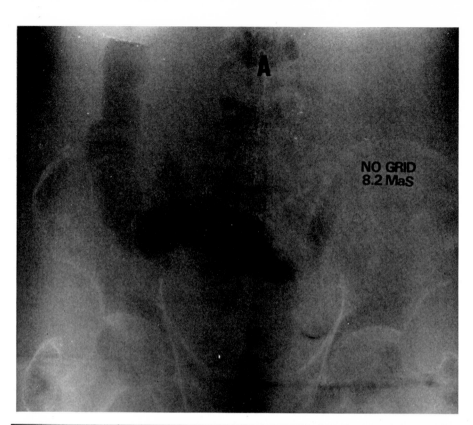

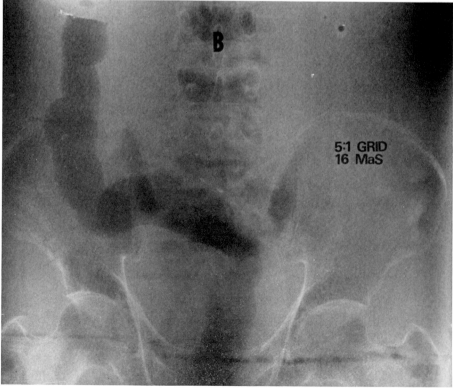

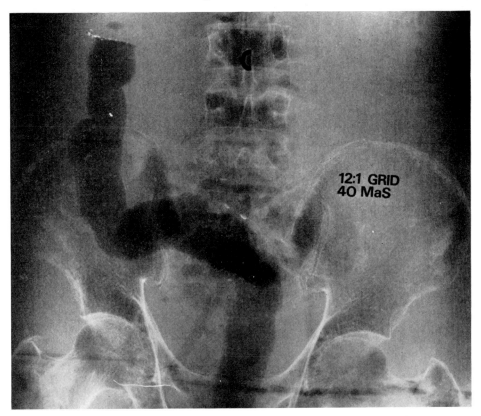

12:1 GRID
40 MaS

← Figure 147. The contrast seen in these films indicates the effect grids have and the importance of proper grid selection. A has virtually no visibility of detail. These radiographs were exposed at 80 KvP.

further summary, grids function on the principle that scatter radiation travels at a more dramatic (divergent) angle as compared to that of the primary photons. Thus, grids allow primary photons to pass through its lead strips easily while "capturing" the more tangent scatter photons and eliminating them from the exposure. Figure 148 illustrates how the lead strips take advantage of this to produce a higher quality image.

Grid Cutoff

With all the absorption of excess scatter radiation by the grid, many of these still manage to get through and reach the film. The primary rays, however, must get to the film's emulsion or a condition known as grid cutoff will result. Grid cutoff is when *too many* primary rays are absorbed by the grid causing areas of decreased density. Figure 149 shows the

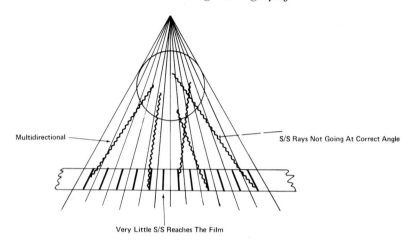

Multidirectional

S/S Rays Not Going At Correct Angle

Very Little S/S Reaches The Film

Figure 148. Scattered photons are trapped by the lead strips.

radiographic effect of grid cutoff. The technologist should be mindful that the degree or amount of lost radiographic density depends on the amount of primary radiation that has been absorbed by the grid.

Grid cutoff can result from a number of conditions which will be discussed later in this chapter; however, it might be beneficial to review Figure 150, which illustrates the two major causes of primary cutoff. Figure 151 shows an improperly positioned focused type grid.

Stereo Radiography

Stereo radiography presents a problem to the technologist with regards to grid cutoff. Figure 152 shows there is no problem in angling the beam along the length of the lead strips; however, it might sometimes be necessary during stereo examinations to angle the beam across the lead strips. The technologist should remember when he shifts across the lead strips that the highest ratio he can successfully use is a 6:1 grid. The reason for this is that if higher ratios are used for *cross grid* shifting, the two stereo radiographs will have unequal densities, and high ratio grids (10:1 and 12:1) would allow no primary photons whatever to reach the film.

High grid ratios do improve radiographic quality and in fact are considered absolutely essential for most x-ray examinations. Because grids are so effective in reducing *excess* amounts of scatter radiation from the remnant beam, they permit the technologist to use higher Kv values. The importance of high KvP exposures in providing decreased patient dose and allowing shorter x-ray exposures to be used should not be taken lightly.

High Ratio Grids and Cutoff

The major disadvantage in using high ratio grids can be seen in Figure 153. From this illustration, you can see that as grid ratio increases, more of the lesser angled rays are eliminated from the remnant beam. It can be imagined, after studying this illustration, that if the ratio is too great not only will the angled S/S rays be removed but too many primary rays will be eliminated from the exposure as well. For this reason, the maximum ratio manufactured for practical use is a 16:1 grid and, as briefly mentioned earlier, these grids have questionable value.

In short, the technologist must choose an appropriate grid ratio which will meet the criteria of (a) providing maximum cleanup and (b) permitting sufficient primary radiation to pass through its lead strips so that cutoff does not occur. A term known as positioning latitude is thus used by technologists to refer to the extent to which a grid can be mispositioned (misaligned with respect to the primary beam) before enough grid cutoff will occur to result in decreased radiographic quality. Grid ratio then controls the amount of positioning latitude (positioning error) a grid will allow. We have been discussing cutoff in terms of high ratio grids; it should be made clear, however, that grid cutoff can also result when using a low grid ratio as well; however, positioning latitude is much greater and repeat exposures are less likely to occur as a result of malalignment between the grid and the primary rays.

Major Types of Grids

There are other important considerations in choosing the correct grid for a particular exposure condition. Grids can be arranged into two *family* groups: liner and cross grids. A linear grid is any grid that has lead strips running in the same direction. A cross grid's lead strips run in opposing directions, usually at 90 degrees to each other. This type of grid forms a "criss-cross pattern" on the radiographic image if inspected closely. Figure 154 shows the two basic designs.

Nonfocused and Focused Grids

The earliest type of grid was the linear grid. For some time this grid seemed more than sufficient; however, as various ideas for new techniques in radiographic procedures were considered and explored, the original linear grid was in need of improvement. The major problem with the linear grid was that it did not allow the remnant beam to pass between its lead strips located at the outer edges of the film. This is because the primary photons coming from the tube are more divergent at the outer beam perimeter as compared to those moving down through the center

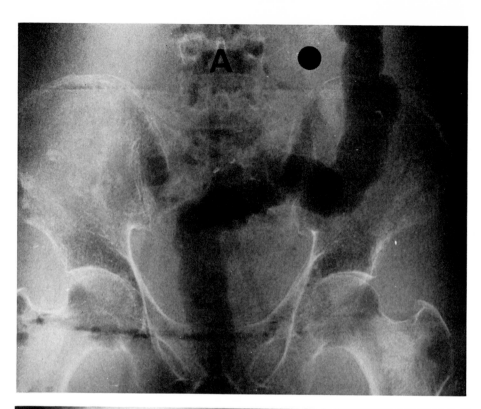

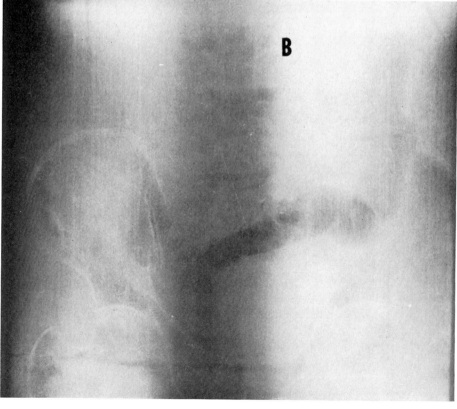

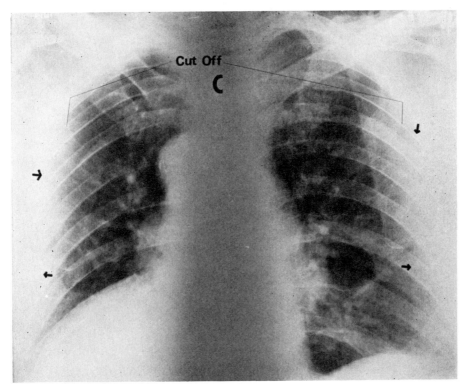

← Figure 149. *A* was exposed using a properly positioned stationary grid. *B* and *C* show the radiographic effect of a poorly positioned grid.

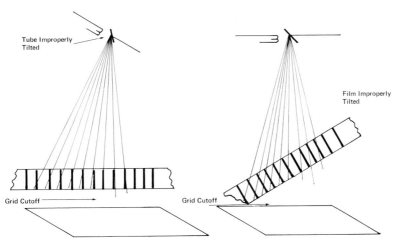

Figure 150. Tube angulation and grid tilt are two very common causes of grid cutoff, especially with portable abdomen or hip examinations. Using the incorrect F.F.D. will also cause serious grid line problems.

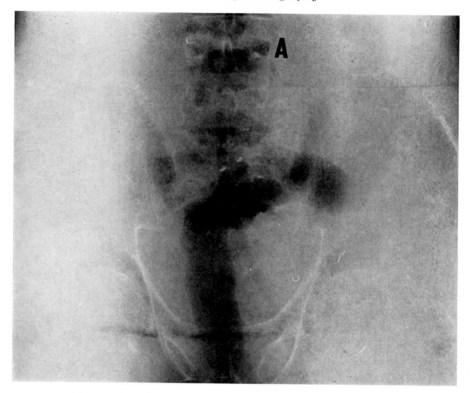

Figure 151. The effect of a focused grid placed upside down.

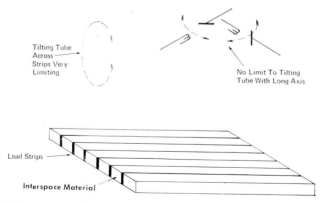

Tilting Tube
Across
Strips Very
Limiting

No Limit To Tilting
Tube With Long Axis

Lead Strips

Interspace Material

Figure 152. Grid stereo radiography poses no problem as long as the tube is angled *with* the lead strips. If the tube is to be shifted across the lead strips, cutoff is likely to occur. Stereo work should not be attempted when cross grids are used.

"core" of the beam. Figure 155 illustrates this situation, the result of which is a marked decrease in radiographic density at the outer edges of the film due to grid cutoff. It must be noted that this condition worsens with (1) shorter focal film distances, (2) large sized films, and (3) with higher grid ratios.

After some reflection on the problem, researchers realized that if the lead strips could be individually angled to varying degrees according to the projected divergence of the primary photons as they pass through the borders of the grid, a more even density distribution would be gained. Figure 156A shows this concept in diagrammatic form. This type of grid became known as a focused grid because its lead strips are "focused" (angled) to accommodate the natural divergence of the primary beam striking the film at the outer edges.

This arrangement was excellent. However, it is necessary to have focused grids made for ranges of focal film distance as noted in Figure 156B. Thus, a focused grid has the important advantage of permitting a uniform passage of primary photons through its lead strips, across the entire surface of the grid. In addition, the focused grid lead strips are indeed "focused" to accommodate the specific divergence which changes according to the focal film distance used. This requires that focused grids be manufactured and used for specific and compatible divergences relative to the focal film distance.

Cross Hatch Grids

With the concept of linear grids (focused and nonfocused) understood, we may now consider the cross grid family which is shown in Figure 154. By definition, the cross hatch grid is basically two linear grids affixed to each other so that the lead strips are at opposing angles. The most common cross grid has the lead strips opposing each other at 90 degrees, however, a rhombic grid has its lead strips opposing each other at 45 degrees.

Like the linear grid, cross grids can be ordered in focused and unfocused types and with a variety of ratios. The major advantage in cross grids is their relatively high cleanup per ratio as compared to linear grids. The major disadvantage regarding cross grids is that they usually cannot be used in a bucky (except for the rhombic design) and that the amount of intentional tube angulation that can be successfully used is very limited. A 5:1 cross grid will have similar positioning latitude to a 5:1 linear grid; but the CR can be angled with the lead strips using a linear grid as much as is desired without risking cutoff while a cross grid does not permit such deliberate angles in any direction. The student should be careful to keep in mind that, whatever design or construction of grid he

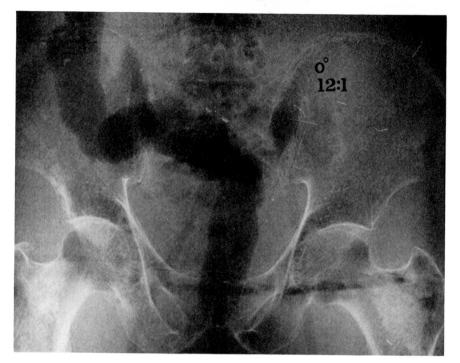

Figure 153A.

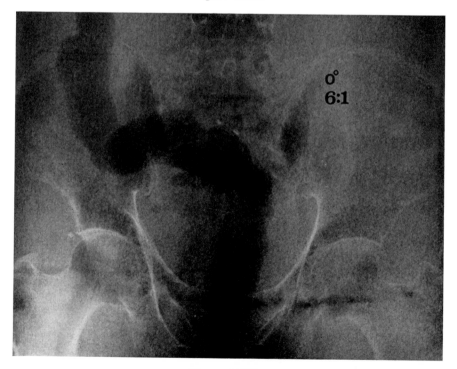

Figure 153B.

Figure 153. As grid ratio increases, the probability of grid cutoff increases.

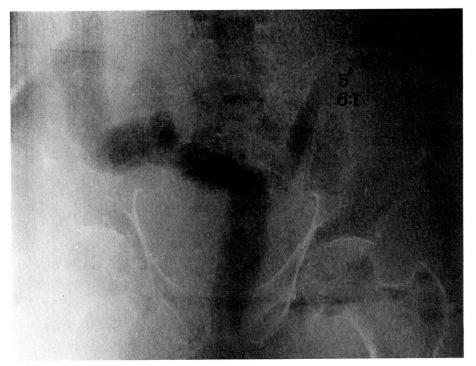

Figure 153C.

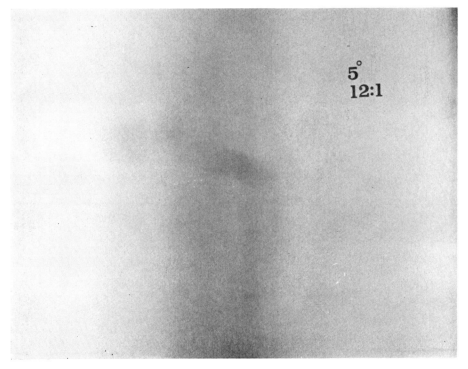

Figure 153D.

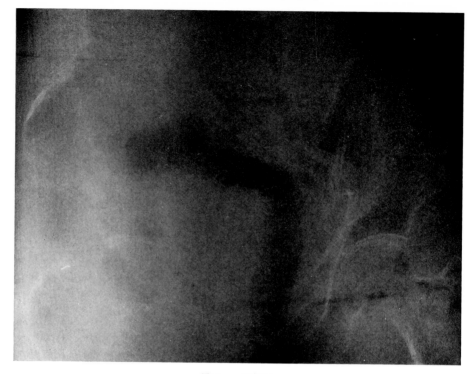

Figure 153E.

chooses, the basic function and rules are always the same regarding positioning latitude, ratio, cleanup, and purpose.

Linear Grid versus Cross Grid

The major advantage of cross grids over linear grids is that cross grids offer better cleanup and equal positioning latitude per ratio than can be expected from the linear grids—providing that deliberate center ray (CR) angulation is not necessary. It is generally accepted that an 8:1 cross grid will approximately equal the efficiency (absorption of S/S) of a 16:1 linear grid, yet the 8:1 cross grid will have wider positioning latitude be-

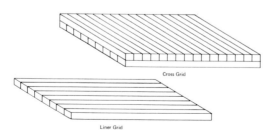

Figure 154.

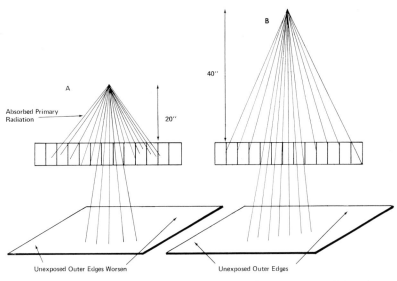

Figure 155. Grid cutoff of this type is the result of an incompatibility between the arrangement of the lead strips and the projected pattern of the photons.

cause of its lower ratio. Figure 157 shows the difference in exposure rates between cross and linear grids and the effect these two grids have on contrast.

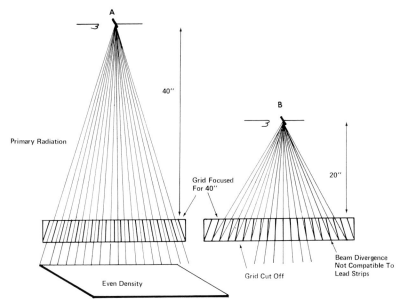

Figure 156. Focused grids are designed in such a way that their lead strips stop the scatter photons but allow the peripheral x-rays to pass through easily. If a focused grid is used when the tube is out of range, grid cutoff will result.

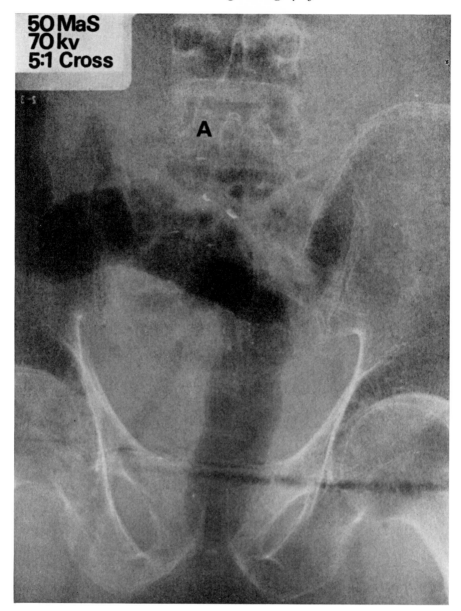

50 MaS
70 kv
5:1 Cross

A

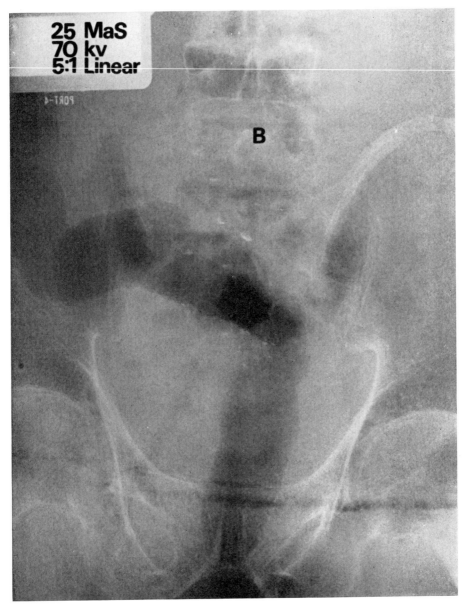

25 MaS
70 kv
5:1 Linear

B

← Figure 157. These radiographs show the effect a cross grid has on the radiographic image compared to a linear grid of equal ratio. Note the exposure values.

Quantity of Lead in the Grid

Earlier in the chapter it was noted that grid ratio is a very important factor in efficiency and cleanup. Yet there is another important contributor to cleanup the technologist should be aware of. It is the factor commonly known as grid weight. It may seem to be a very basic point, but the quality of lead used (purity) to make the lead strips plays an important role in a grid's absorbing ability. The main idea to keep in mind here is that as long as lead content (type of grid weight) is consistent, the ratio will determine cleanup, and as a rule, grid manufacturers maintain a relatively uniform lead composition.

Moving Grids

A bucky assembly is a device that was invented in 1920 to put the conventional linear grid in motion during the x-ray exposure. The advantage in moving a grid during the exposure is that the grid lines can be totally blurred and made invisible in the radiographic image.

A similar effect will result if a photograph is taken of a fast moving object. The faster and smaller the object is, the closer it comes to becoming invisible on the photograph as a result of the blurring effect. With grids, the lead strips are very thin; when put in motion by the bucky, they become invisible in the radiographic image.

In general, bucky assemblies are used with focused grids. With the use of modern high capacity generators, technologists now have the option of using very short exposures, which is almost always an important advantage. However, very short exposures can complicate the use of a bucky assembly somewhat. The problem with fast exposures and bucky assemblies is that occasionally the exposure is so fast that it actually radiographs the grid in motion resulting in grid lines on the film. To correct this situation another breed of grid was designed and has become known as a fine line or micro line grid, which will be discussed later in the chapter. A fine line grid does not have to move during the exposure which permits the technologist to use the shortest exposure he wishes without fear of obvious grid lines.

Types of Bucky Assemblies

There are two major types of bucky assemblies: reciprocating and reciprocatic. The difference is that the reciprocating bucky moves at two different speeds during the exposure and that the reciprocatic bucky moves at one speed. The motion of the reciprocatic bucky is somewhat faster and thus allows slightly shorter exposures to be used without producing grid lines. These bucky assemblies push and pull a grid sideways under the table during the exposure. The total distance moved to either side of center while the grid is in motion is approximately one inch. The excursion of the grid from side to side causes a slight degree of decentering (see Fig. 158) and, as might be expected from such a situation, additional absorption of the primary beam occurs. For this reason, bucky exposures taken with equal grid ratios and lead content will produce slightly less radiographic density than if the same grid was exposed as a stationary grid.

In summary, one can say that grids can be used in one of two ways, stationary and moving. Stationary grids are used mainly for portable and operating room radiography, and occasionally in the radiographic room for various cross table studies. The bucky is used in all table x-ray work except for body parts that measure more than 10 cm and for a small number of special techniques, such as radiography of the paranasal sinuses. The use of a bucky assembly partially determines the standard focal film distance for table work. Because a certain amount of space is necessary for the bucky to function in its place between the film and the under side of the table, object film distance is inevitable. As discussed in Chapter Six, object film distance causes magnification and increases penumbra, but increasing the focal film distance can reduce this problem somewhat. The focal film distance has thus been set at 40 inches to minimize the approximate 2.5 inches of object film distance needed for the bucky. Previous to this, focal film distances were commonly 36 inches.

GRIDS AND THE GENERAL RADIOGRAPHIC EFFECT

Radiographic Density

The radiographic effect can be seen in two forms, density and contrast. Density is affected greatly because so much scatter radiation which had previously reached and exposed the film is now removed from the remnant beam. In addition, small amounts of primary radiation are absorbed by the grid. Contrast is affected because fog caused by S/S radiation is greatly eliminated. In general, 55 percent of the density of a chest exposure and approximately 90 percent of the radiographic density of an abdomen film is caused by S/S radiation. This means that for a chest examination only 45 percent of the density is caused by the primary beam and for an abdomen examination only 10 percent of the radiographic density is caused by the primary beam. If we consider the fact that a 12:1 ratio grid will eliminate up to 95 percent of the S/S radiation from the beam, we begin to appreciate how important the use of grids really is. Figure 159 shows two radiographs exposed with different grid ratios.

There is some question among technologists as to whether it is proper

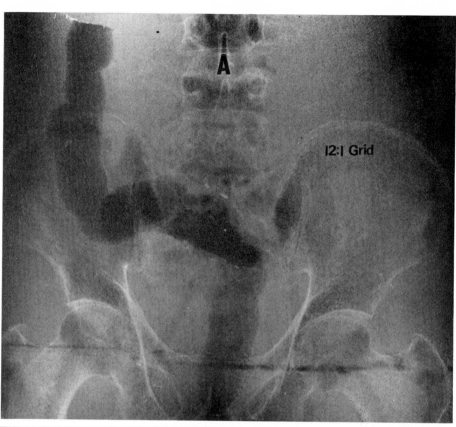

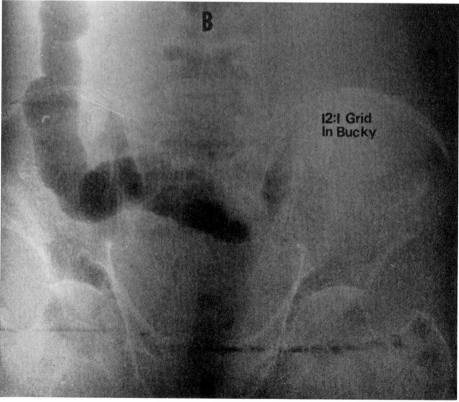

to increase KvP to compensate for the decreased density caused by grids. Although both methods are used, the author prefers increases in MaS. The reason for this is that grids are, after all, used primarily to improve radiographic contrast while absorbing excessive amounts of S/S radiation from the remnant beam. The adjustments needed for additional exposure is only to gain back the lost density, and increasing MaS performs this function very well. On the other hand, if Kv is used to regain the lost radiographic density when a 12:1 grid is used, an increase of approximately 20 to 26 KvP is required. When radiographing a moderate to thick body part, an increase of this magnitude would cause a substantial amount of additional scatter. Thus, if the 95 percent of S/S is removed by the 12:1 grid but the technologist compensates for the loss in radiographic density by increasing 20 to 26 KvP, the net effect of the grid in increasing contrast has been seriously compromised. Another argument against using KvP to compensate for different grid ratios is that the contrast media used for various examinations has an optimum KvP absorption rate. For example, the contrast manufactured by a major pharmaceutical company for doing IVP examinations often recommends a KvP that is not higher than 75. It might be helpful to recap the important results that use of grids have on the radiographic image. Please note the statement below:

As grid ratio increases absorption of excessive S/S photons increases causing less S/S to expose the film. This, in turn, provides for a higher radiographic contrast.

Selecting the Proper Grid

The fact that there is a wide selection implies no one grid will perform optimally under all conditions. The determining factors for the purpose of grid selection are derived by considering two major conditions. The first is how much S/S will be produced with a given kilovoltage and body part, and the second is the environment in which the grid ratio will be used. It is advisable to study these major factors separately.

Scatter Radiation

The amount of S/S radiation produced as a result of interactions between the primary photons and the body tissues has already been adequately discussed: The primary influencing factor in S/S production is KvP and the makeup of the body part being radiographed.

KILOVOLTAGE: Kilovoltage has an important effect on the ratio of S/S

← Figure 158. Note the density differences in A and B. Published figures from Liebel Flarsheim Corporation indicate a 20 percent density variation between stationary grid and bucky work. *Courtesy of* Liebel Flarsheim Corporation, Cincinnati, Ohio.

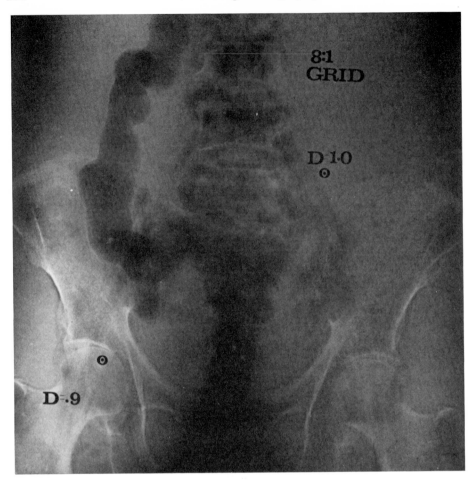

to primary radiation that is produced during an exposure. (It is the ratio of primary and scatter rays in the remnant beam that determines whether fog will result on the radiographic image.) The proper kilovoltage level is determined principally by atomic number, thickness, and body part density. An average lateral lumbar spine exposure requires the use of higher kilovoltages than an average shoulder or knee examination. Not all radiologists and technologists agree on the precise KvP level. However, there is usually general agreement that as the body part's atomic number and density increases, the KvP also should be increased.

One major decision that the technologist must make is to choose the proper grid ratio. The technologist should also keep in mind the major function of a grid is to clean up excessive scatter radiation from the remnant beam and, of course, the primary determinant in cleanup is grid ratio. Since scatter-producing interactions increase rapidly with increases in KvP above 70, more "grid" is necessary to absorb the additional scatter photons. Figure 160 gives a suggested KvP and grid ratio combination. In short, KvP has a strong bearing on the ratio that is to be used be-

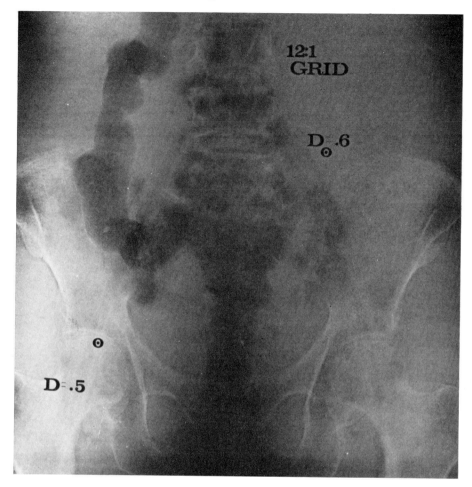

← Figure 159. As grid ratio increases radiographic density decreases, primarily because the scattered photons that would otherwise reach the film and add density are absorbed by the lead strips. Some additional primary photons are also absorbed.

cause Kv strongly influences the type of interactions that will be produced by the body. As KvP increases over 70, disproportionately greater amounts of Compton interactions result as compared to photoelectric interactions; it is the Compton interactions that account for the amount of S/S production that causes fog.

BODY PART: Patient thickness and density also strongly influence the overall amount of S/S radiation the body will ultimately emit. As discussed earlier, patient thickness and tissue density vary with body habitus, body part, and pathology. However, to reiterate, scatter radiation increases with body thickness and tissue density. As one can imagine, it would be extremely impractical for the technologist to change the grid ratio for every patient with different body thicknesses and density, so practically all x-ray tables have one type of grid installed. The most common type of grid in modern installations is a 12:1 ratio focused at 40 inches.

GRID SELECTION ON BASIS OF CLEANUP REQUIREMENTS				
Cleanup	Type	Positioning Latitude	Recommended Up To	Remarks
SUPERLATIVE	6:1 Criss-cross	Good	110 KVP	Tube tilt limited to five degrees.
EXCELLENT	12:1 Linear	Very slight	110 KVP (Suitable for higher kilo-voltages)	Extra care required for proper alignment; usually used in fixed mount.
	5:1 Criss-cross	Extreme	100 KVP	Tube tilt limited to five degrees.
VERY GOOD	10:1 Linear	Slight	100 KVP	Reasonable care required for proper alignment.
GOOD	8:1 Linear	Fair	100 KVP	For general stationary grid use.
MODERATE	6:1 Linear 5:1 Linear	Extreme	80 KVP	Very easy to use.

Figure 160. *Courtesy of* Liebel Flarsheim Corporation.

The Environment

The technologist must be equally careful when choosing a particular grid depending on the environment in which the examination is to be accomplished. The term "environment" is used here to describe the conditions under which the exposure is to be made, for example, whether the exposure will be in the patient's room using portable equipment, in the operating room, or in the radiographic room for cross-table exposures.

Without question, the key idea for the technologist to keep in mind during such potentially troublesome situations is the amount of positioning latitude the grid he will choose has to offer. As was pointed out earlier, positioning latitude is dependent largely on grid ratio. The perfect grid under any circumstance would be one that has very wide positioning latitude and very good cleanup. Unfortunately, these are mutually exclusive characteristics because high grid ratios are used for superior cleanup and efficiency and wide positioning latitude can only be gained with low ratio grid. From the radiographs shown earlier, it was noted how much of the image can be lost because of improper positioning of the grid. It is here that the greatest compromise in grid selection must be made. Because of the high probability of grid cutoff occurring when high grid ratios are used for the less than ideal exposure environment, cleanup is usually sacrificed for practicality. With this in mind, a 5:1 or 6:1 ratio is usually the most popular choice.

Even a "routine" portable hip examination can turn out to be a nightmare of unnecessary repeats if the grid used offers too little positioning latitude. Through experience, it will become painfully clear that if a light radiograph is obtained and the cause of the light film is improperly diagnosed as underexposed, additional trouble is close at hand. For example, the author has seen student technologists too quickly guess that their portable abdomen film was too light because they did not use enough exposure. For the repeat film they doubled the exposure, but as luck would have it, the grid was positioned properly for the second exposure and, to their amazement, the repeat film was now too dark. This meant that they had to take a third film. To make matters worse, it is standard procedure at this point to claim the portable unit is not working properly, leaving the whole situation in that much more disarray (see Fig. 161). To reduce the possibilities of this occurring, it is the author's opinion that technologists should use a grid not greater than 6:1 for portable or operating room work. (A 5:1 grid absorbs approximately 80% of the scatter and a 6:1 absorbs approximately 85% of scatter [see Fig. 162].)

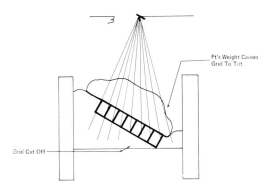

Figure 161. It is difficult for the technologist to see how the grid is aligned with the CR under these conditions, but an intuition can be developed with experience.

If circumstances make maximum cleanup esssential, a low ratio (5:1) cross grid is suggested. Because of their construction, cross grids produce unusually high cleanup per grid ratio. To some extent cross grids do offer the best of two worlds. A 5:1 cross grid will provide the cleanup equal to a 10:1 linear grid, yet because of its low ratio it has wide positioning latitude. The drawback to using cross grids, as was mentioned earlier, is that deliberate angles of center ray cannot be accomplished successfully.

FOCAL FILM DISTANCE: Focal distance should also be taken into account when choosing grids for a particular purpose. During earlier discussions on focus grids, it was emphasized that although grids are not focused for a *specific* focal distance, like 37 or 42 inches, they are limited to *ranges of* focal distances. For example, a grid rated for use at 40 inches can also successfully be used at 35 to 50 inches. When a focused grid is used at a wrong focal film distance, cutoff occurs and is most likely to show itself at the edges of the film (see Fig. 149C). As higher grid ratios

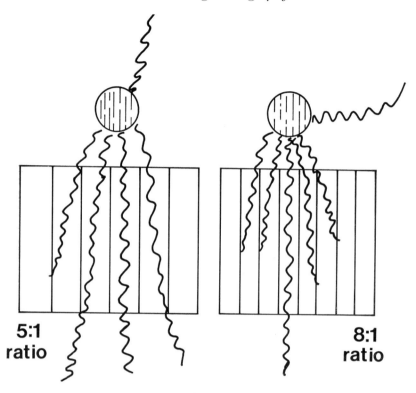

5:1 ratio

8:1 ratio

Figure 162. Compare the placement of the lead strips between the 5:1 and the 8:1 ratio grids. Because of this important factor, the 8:1 grid will allow fewer S/S rays to reach the film and contrast increase as density will decrease. Positioning latitude decreases with the 8:1 ratio grid in this illustration.

are used under these improper conditions, cutoff will worsen. Larger film sizes will also cause this problem to worsen. Parallel grids should be used at the longest focal film distance possible to avoid this peripheral grid cutoff condition. The reason for this is that the lead strips are perfectly vertical, and using increased focal film distances tends to produce a beam whose photons are approaching the film at a more vertical plane.

Chest radiography requires a grid with slightly different construction characteristics than those noted above. A very important factor in good chest radiography is to use the shortest exposure time possible. Because of this, a bucky assembly would be of no real value, since the very rapid exposures (one-sixtieth of a second and less) would radiograph the grid in motion resulting in visible grid lines on the film. To avoid this, bucky assemblies were abandoned altogether and a special grid with very finely cut lead strips (usually 100 to 110 lines per inch) was substituted. These fine line grids have the same basic design as the conventional grids previously discussed, except the lead strips and interspace materials are cut very thin. For example, a standard grid has between 60 and 80 lead strips (lines) per inch so that they can be relatively thick, but these produce a rather obvious distraction to the radiologist when viewing a number of films per day because the lead strips are so visible. With regard to fine line grids, to fit 100 to 110 lines per inch the lead strip has to be extremely thin—when radiographed the lead lines are virtually invisible at normal viewing distances even though this grid is not moving during the exposure. The obvious choice for a grid in chest radiography would be of a high ratio because most often high KvPs (over 100) are used. A desirable installation for chest radiography would be a 12:1 ratio grid focused at 72 inches with 110 lines per inch.

As important as it is for the technologist to use higher grid ratios with high KvP values in thick, dense body parts, it is important to remember to reduce ratio when lower KvPs are used. If this general rule is not followed, the lower penetrating beam will not have sufficient energy to pass through the high ratio grid and unusually high radiographic contrast will result because of underpenetration. To prevent this from happening, students should keep in mind the x-ray beam must not only penetrate the patient adequately but also penetrate the grid as well.

GRID CASSETTES: Grid cassettes are used as a matter of convenience. In a busy department, it is a nuisance to tape and untape stationary grids to cassettes. However, grid cassettes are very expensive, and because a large number of grid cassettes would be needed for a department, there is justifiable reluctance to purchase any more than necessary. In construction, a grid cassette is a standard cassette of any size with a grid built into the bakelite. Any kind of grid design can be purchased as a grid cassette.

SUMMARY

We often become frustrated when there are so few standards and constants for choosing proper exposure conditions including grids. Categorical answers come hard in the medical field because the end result is so dependent upon the patient who can, and usually does, provide an extremely wide range of variables with which we are expected to work. For this reason, it is often best for the student to understand well the various *concepts* surrounding a particular problem before any attempt is made toward a solution.

There is no one grid type, Kv level, body habitus, type of film, or processing condition that will work equally well for all conditions, and it is up to the technologist to make the final decision correctly by evaluating the particular exposure problem at hand.

CHAPTER TEN

TOMOGRAPHY

THROUGHOUT THE AUTHOR's own experience, tomography has proved to be both an interesting challenge and a very beneficial diagnostic tool. In recent years much more sophisticated equipment has been made available with startlingly improved radiographic results. These more complicated units as well as the more simply designed tomographic units will be discussed along with their relative values later in the chapter. We should first look closely at some of the basic concepts involved in tomography. The terms "tomography," "planography," and "body section" are all synonyms and are thus often used interchangeably.

WHY DO WE USE TOMOGRAPHY?

The purpose of tomography is to make visible those structures that are not clearly seen radiographically because of their location in the body. Very often structures of interest are located beneath very dense body parts and can therefore not be seen by conventional radiography. Figure 163 compares a few tomograms made at crucial levels compared with routine radiographs of the same area. There is no specific organ or body part that may not be tomographed. Virtually any area of the body can be successfully "cut," as long as it has some reasonable thickness and the specific body part under examination is somewhat poorly visualized by surrounding structures. The cervical spine is an excellent example of a thin structure that is very successfully tomographed. The inner ear is perhaps one of the most difficult structures to demonstrate by conventional radiography, but can be nicely demonstrated with the use of tomography. It is easy to understand the value of tomography after reviewing these radiographs.

The Basic Concept

The importance of immobilizing the patient to prevent blurring is obvious. When the patient is allowed to move a body part under examination during the exposure a marked decrease in sharpness results, but motion can be occasionally used to the technologist's advantage. Tomog-

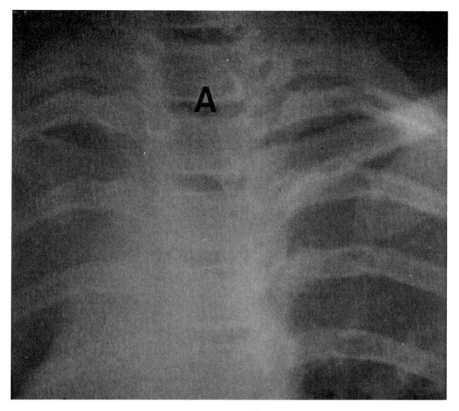

Figure 163A.

Figure 163. These radiographs show the value of tomography over conventional radiography when superimposed body structures are to be demonstrated.

raphy puts to use the concept that motion makes body structures invisible by blurring. During a tomographic study, an attempt is made to selectively blur unwanted structures while maintaining sharpness of the specific body part under examination. With tomography, the motion is not generated by the patient but rather by the x-ray equipment. In Figure 164, a metal rod has been drawn and accompanied by arrows showing its tilting motion. The arrows indicate motion along its entire length except at the pivot point. This point will be referred to henceforth as the fulcrum. If an x-ray tube is attached to one end of the rod and a film to the other end, we can begin to see something that resembles a functional tomographic mechanism (see Fig. 165). If a patient is placed as illustrated, one can begin to see that motion will occur at all levels of the body except at the fulcrum. If the technologist is using equipment that provides a method by which the fulcrum can be raised or lowered at will, virtually any level of the body can be made visible while all other structures lying

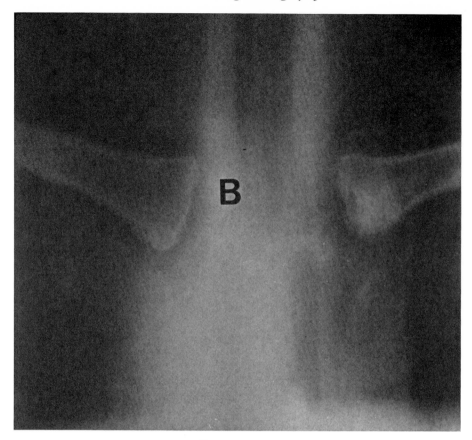

Figure 163B.

outside *that plane* will be practically invisible. Thus, it is the fulcrum that establishes the objective plane so that a specific level of the body can be tomographed. It should be pointed out that the area of clarity is not limited to the fulcrum point alone, but to the entire horizontal plane extending from each side of the fulcrum. Hence, all structures lying at the level of the fulcrum will be of equal sharpness. In short, the purpose of tomography is to improve visibility of specific body parts of interest that are surrounded by other body parts. The increased visibility is accomplished by deliberate blurring of all structures lying above and below the objective plane.

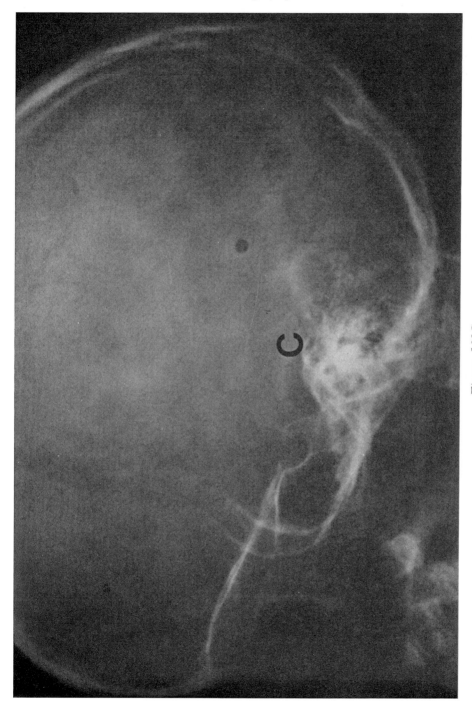

Figure 163C.

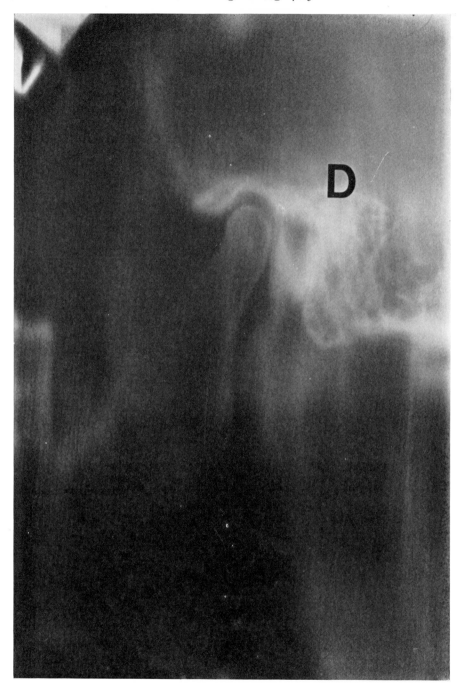

Figure 163D.

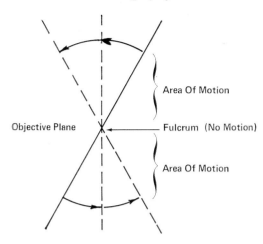

Figure 164. The basic concept of the fulcrum and resulting objective plane.

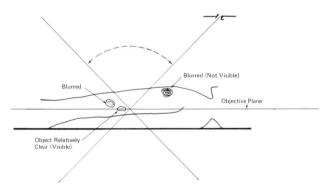

Figure 165. The basic components of a tomographic unit: a pivot point (fulcrum), a connecting shaft holding the tube and film in place, the x-ray tube, and bucky.

MAKING ADJUSTMENTS FOR CUT THICKNESS

There is another dimension to the objective plane—thickness. It is necessary that thickness of the objective plane be changed from time to time and this is handled quite easily by controlling the distance the tube travels *during the exposure.* In reviewing Figure 166, one can see that the area of sharpness (the objective plane) becomes thicker as the excursion of the tube decreases. The distance the tube travels *during the exposure* is known as arc. A very short arc, such as 10°, would produce a thick objective plane (cut) known as a zonogram, whereas a 50° arc would produce a very thin cut. Figure 167 shows a zonogram of a kidney compared with a cut made using a 50° arc. The value of zonography is that, if done properly, an entire organ or at least a large part of a structure can be seen as a unit on the film, as opposed to seeing the structure in

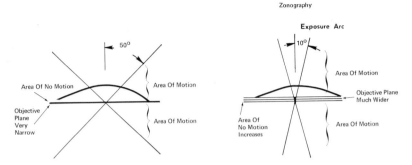

Figure 166. A 10 degree arc is commonly used for doing zonography. It is the exposure arc (the arc of the tube *during* the exposure), not the total distance the tube travels, that determines thickness of the objective plane.

many separate radiographic slices. As a result, the composition of the zonogram structure can be seen with more continuity. Often, zonograms of the kidney are obtained during a drip infusion study. On the other hand, it is common to use very thin cuts for x-ray examinations of small intricate bony structures as well as for bone examinations, and tomograms of the inner and middle ear region are often accomplished with a 40 or 50 degree arc.

In summary, not only the level of an intended cut can be adjusted by raising or lowering the height of the fulcrum but the thickness of the cut can be adjusted as well by changing the FFD providing this adjustment in FFD will cause the exposure arc to change also. The greater the arc the thinner the objective plane will become, and vice versa. Figure 168 shows that changing the FFD will not necessarily change the exposure arc depending on the unit being used. Because the general rule of beam geometry holds regarding FFD, short focal film distances for tomography are seldom, if ever, used. In fact, many feel a 48 inch FFD is optimal for obtaining image sharpness.

EXCURSION SPEED

Excursion speed may be described as the quickness with which the tube and film move during the exposure. There is no relationship between excursion speed and the level or thickness of the objective plane. There is, as you might expect, a direct relationship between excursion speed and exposure time. With the more simplified tomographic equipment, there is a series of switches located under the table and arranged in such a way to both initiate and terminate an exposure (shown in Fig. 169). Clearly, if the excursion speed is set by the technologist to be fast, the exposure will be short because the x-ray tube will pass the on and off switches more quickly.

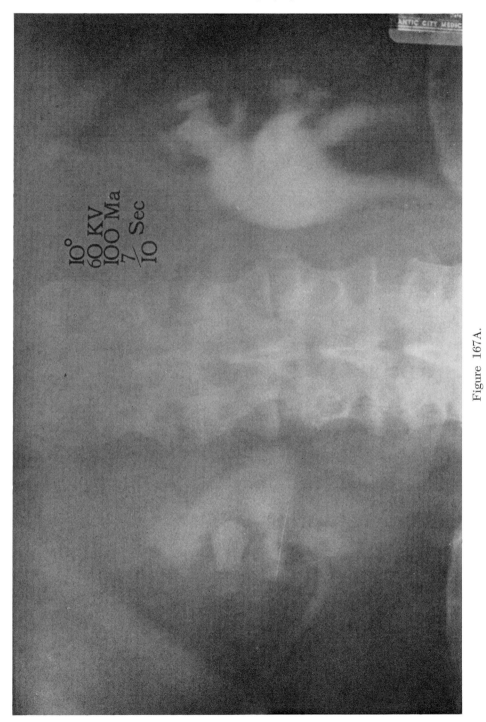

Figure 167A.

Figure 167. These three radiographs compare cut thickness. Note the indicated exposure values.

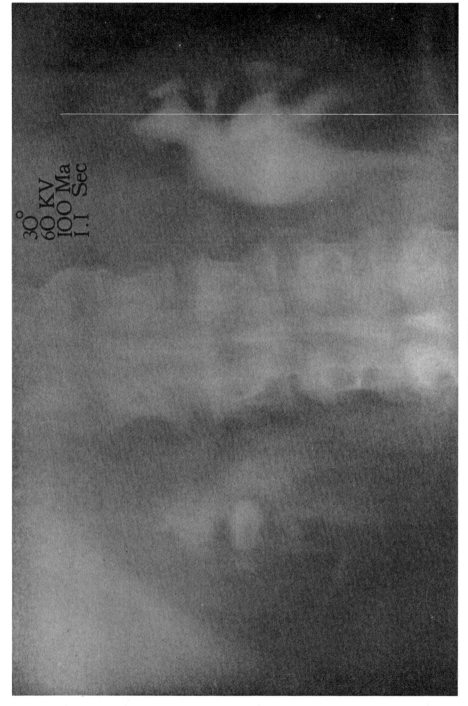

30°
60 KV
100 Ma
1.1 Sec

Figure 167B.

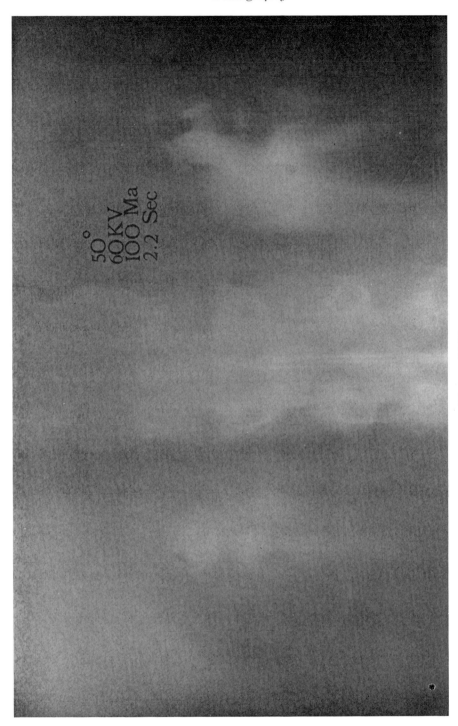

Figure 167C.

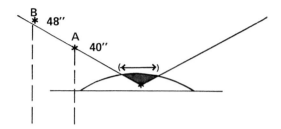

Figure 168.

Although intentional motion is vital to tomography, only certain movements are permitted. The term "unstable linkage" is used here to describe any situation that would allow unwanted motion of the tube or film. Poor (unstable) linkage most often occurs with lightweight equipment common to dual purpose units. Such units if properly calibrated, however, can produce good results, but if they are used improperly, important stress points in the tube and bucky drive mechanism soon begin to give way and loosen. If this process continues, sharpness of the objective plane will decrease resulting in a slow erosion of tomographic quality.

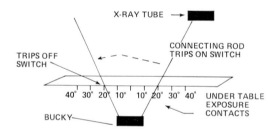

Figure 169. Although this design is certainly not a standard among manufacturers, it illustrates that the technologist does not initiate the *actual* exposure and that the x-ray tube usually travels some distance before the exposure begins.

Poor linkage can be seen radiographically in the form of excessive smearing and unsharpness of the objective plane, but because there is always some blurring present on the tomographic image it is difficult or impossible to tell how much is from "natural" causes and how much is the result of loose mechanical connections. Figure 170 shows a typical dual-purpose, lightweight tomographic unit compared to one of more substantial and sophisticated design.

Figure 171 shows schematically the type of excess motion that commonly results from unstable linkage. Three points might be valuable to consider in attempting to reduce unnecessary tube motion. (1) Use a slow speed for the majority of radiographic work and especially for cutting

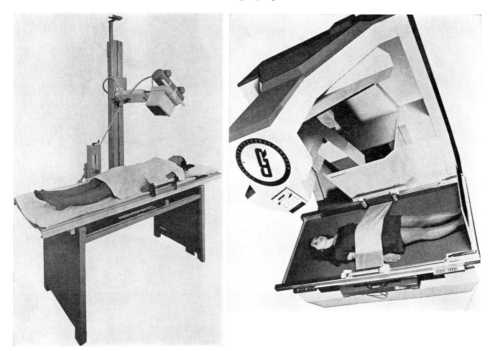

Figure 170. The variation in tomographic equipment design. *Courtesy of* C.G.R. Corporation.

small, difficult to visualize body parts. If the tube moves too quickly through its excursion there is what appears to be a jerking motion initially from which the tube has difficulty recovering as it moves over the patient. Often the tube will still be wobbling slightly after it has made contact with the first turn-on switch. (2) Be sure all knobs that are to be loosened are properly loosened so that once in motion, the tube and film can continue without unnecessary resistance. Any friction or resistance between moving parts can give rise to an unsmooth tube film excursion resulting in decreased image sharpness. (3) Place the body part under examination as close to the film as possible. There is some feeling, incorrectly held by technologists, that the rule of using the shortest objective film distance possible does not apply in tomography, however, this is not the case.

TYPES OF EXCURSION PATTERNS

As long as the prerequisites for a smooth tube film excursion are met (movement without wobbling, jerking, etc.) during the exposure, a more complex excursion pattern will yield less smear and streaking of the tomographic image. With this in mind, manufacturers have designed tomographic equipment that will move in a rather complicated pattern. Figure

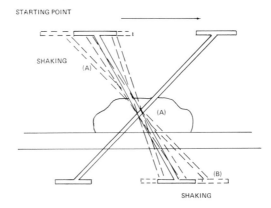

Figure 171. This type of unstable linkage can cause image blurring of the objective plane. When this cannot be corrected mechanically, longer exposure times are advised to reduce tube speed.

172 shows tracings of motions that have become commonplace in modern tomography.

The simplest motion is known as "linear." Although it is still one of the most often used, it does not produce the quality of structure visibility as does the more complex patterns. The problem with linear tomography is that it produces an excess of streaks and smearing that are longitudinal to the direction of the tube motion (see Fig. 173). It can be seen that such blurring certainly detracts from both the overall appearance of the image and more importantly its diagnostic value. This streaking occurs at the points immediately above and below the objective plane as noted in Figure 174. It might be of interest to note that with thin to very thin cuts, these striations will usually appear more pronounced when compared to

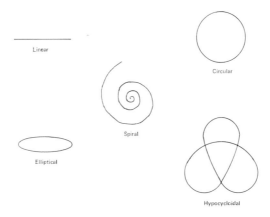

Figure 172. Tracings of commonly used tomographic excursion patterns.

tomographs made with thicker cuts. One way to reduce this type of excess blurring is to arrange the body part so that the long axis of the structure under examination is diagonal and preferably perpendicular to the direction of tube motion (Fig. 175). Figure 176 compares images produced with linear and elliptical patterns. A notable decrease in streaking can be seen as the tube pattern becomes more complex. These more complex excursion patterns are very valuable, especially for the smaller complex structures such as the inner ear.

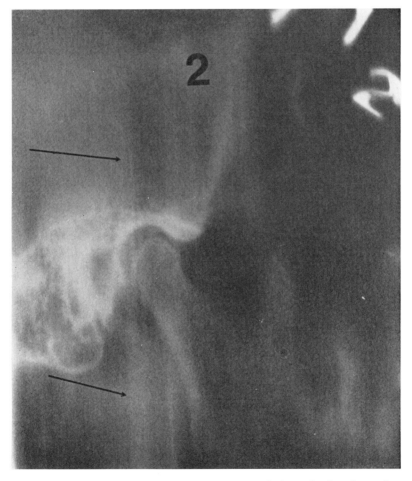

Figure 173. This streaking (also called redundant and ghost shadows) can become so noticeable and obvious it obscures the structures lying in the objective plane.

THE BOOK CASSETTE AND MULTIPLANOGRAPHY

All tomographic equipment has adjustable fulcrum heights as noted earlier. However, a method is available that produces more than one

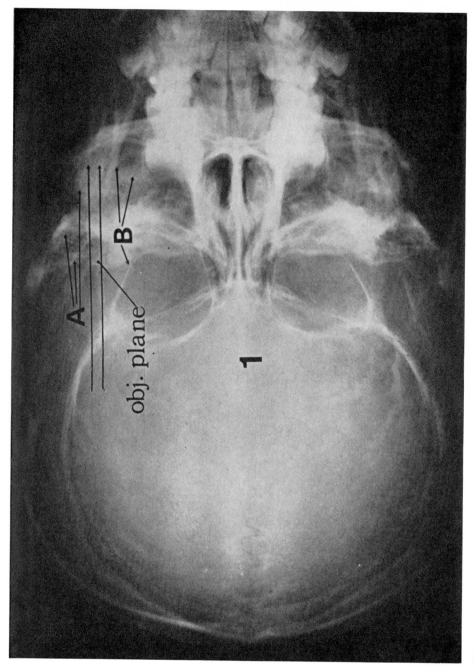

Figure 174. A skull in the lateral position. As the beam is passing through this body part (t.m. joint), other *prominent* body structures are projected to the film as well. These prominent structures are not totally blurred because they are so close to the border of the objective plane.

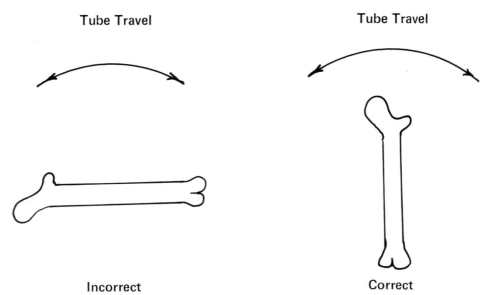

Figure 175. For linear tomography, the body part should be positioned with its long axis in such a way that the tube *will not* move parallel to it.

objective plane with a single exposure. This is known as multiplanography and has questionable value for two important reasons. (1) A device called a book cassette is used (as noted in Fig. 177) which is very thick and causes a great increase in object film distance. It is composed of as many as seven individual sets of intensifying screens that are arranged to be 0.5 to 1 cm apart. The object film distance caused by the thickness of this cassette ranges anywhere from 2.5 inches for the first film to 5 inches for the film that is at the bottom of the cassette. (2) Because the beam loses a moderate amount of intensity as it reaches the film stacked at the bottom of the cassette, it is necessary that the bottom few screens have fast speed screens, and this, of course, decreases sharpness of detail even further.

The combination of these two factors has resulted in decreased interest of multiplanography because of the lack of sharpness. The advantage of multiplanography is that it is a very quick way to produce many different levels of the body part with one exposure. Thus, it can be used effectively as a scanning tool by which approximate levels or structures can be located. Once the structure is located, conventional tomography could be used for the final diagnostic cuts. Thus, the trial and error procedure for finding the correct level of a body part would be greatly reduced and there would be a significant decrease in patient dose as well. Multiplanography is not a popular technique today.

Plesiotomography utilizes the same book cassette concept but it is

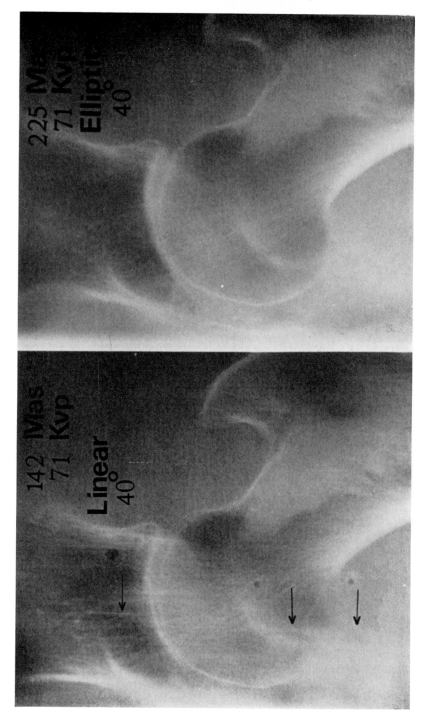

Figure 176. As the pattern of tube motion becomes more complex, ghost or redundant shadows are reduced or eliminated.

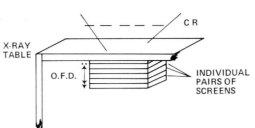

Figure 177. A book cassette as designed and used, revealing one of its most important disadvantages—increased O.F.D.

much thinner and mainly used for radiographing smaller parts such as the middle ear. The standard book cassette noted above commonly produces cuts 1 or 0.5 cm apart, whereas the plesiotomography cassette produces cuts approximately 1 mm apart. Also, there are usually only three or four films used in the plesiotomography cassette as compared to seven with the standard book cassette. More recently, tomographic equipment has been used in conjunction with special procedures, but the expense of this equipment restricts its practical use in many departments.

THICK VERSUS THIN CUTS

The technologist and radiologist have an important option when doing tomography work that can mean the difference between a study of optimal quality or something considerably less. It involves the choice of whether thick or thin cuts are to be obtained. It has been the author's experience that diffuse, loosely constructed structures are often better visualized when moderate to thick cuts are used. However, better results can be noted if dense and unevenly constructed body parts are cut thinly. If a dense but thin body part, such as bone, is to be examined, a thick or thin cut may be used to produce excellent visibility. When equipment that is not of the sophisticated multipattern design is used for too thin a cut, the results are often unsuccessful because the zone of semisharpness which lies immediately above and below the objective plane dominates the visibility of the structures of the objective plane. The result of this is an image with excessive amount of streaking and little structural detail. With multidirectional equipment, however, thin cuts can be made with much less streaking, thereby allowing the objective plane to dominate the image instead of vice versa.

ZONOGRAPHY

Zonography is the technique using tomography equipment that produces a very thick cut on the order of 6.5 cm, as compared to 1.19 mm which is commonly used in routine work. Zonograms are important be-

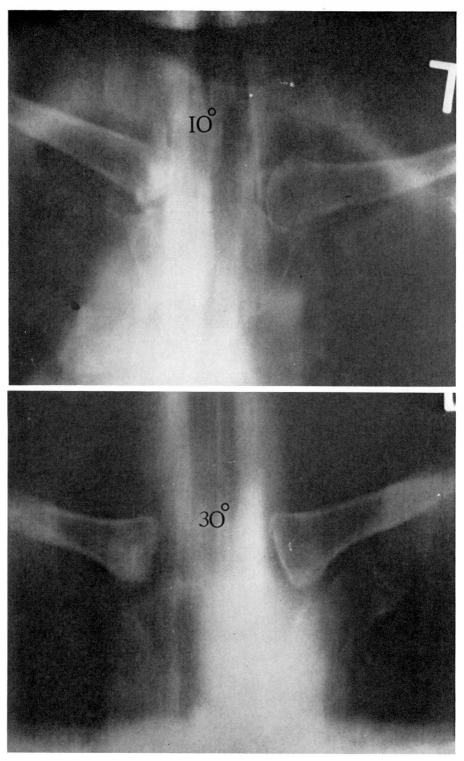

Figure 178. Thick cuts have important advantages over thin cuts when the structure under examination is to be viewed as a consolidated unit.

cause they can produce such a thick cut that often the entire body part under examination would be included in the objective plane. Zonograms are accomplished, as noted earlier, by using a short exposure arc or amplitude. A popular arc used for this function is 10°. Figure 178 shows the effect that zonography has on visualizing a body part compared to other exposure arcs.

CHOOSING A STARTING POINT

Nothing can be more frustrating to the technologist if he cannot locate the body part tomographically and the book cassette is not available. To begin with, no attempt at tomography should be made until an adequate set of routine films are obtained. To find a structure in a patient's chest, for example, the first thing to do is to place the patient properly on the table keeping in mind that the body part to be planographed should be as close to the table as possible. The reason for this, of course, is to maximize sharpness of detail by reducing the object film distance. Oblique positions can also be helpful in this regard. A pair of calipers can be used to localize the level of the structure to be tomographed (see Fig. 179). If properly marked and if the tomographic unit is cutting at the level indicated on the scale, such a device can be used quickly and easily to avoid wasted time in taking many unnecessary scout films. This type of localizer is used for mainly palpable structures, however. A good knowledge of topographic anatomy aids greatly in estimating the position of internal body structures.

For planograming of structures set deep within the chest or abdomen, "eyeballing" the routine film is the only alternative. Figure 180 shows how this can be done effectively: Such measurements are approximate because there is at least a moderate amount of shifting of internal structures between the time the patient is standing for an erect chest, for example, than when he is in a recumbent position on the tomographic table. Also

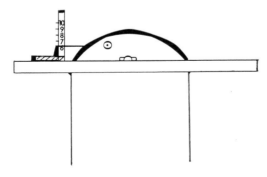

Figure 179.

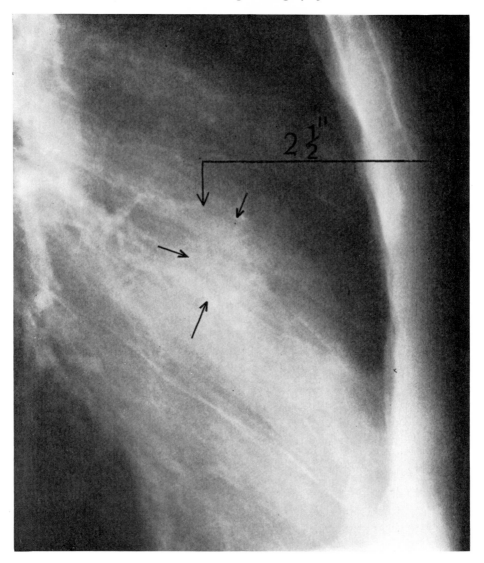

keep in mind that the patient's breathing motion should be stopped for each tomographic exposure made. There is a common practice to simply have the patient stop breathing immediately upon command, but the command is sometimes given at different points of the patient's breathing. The problem with this, of course, is that it takes only little differences in phases of respiration to affect the immediate position of a structure such as a calcified node in the chest or perhaps a duct system of the gall-bladder.

The patient's comfort should be an important consideration from both a professional point of view and a technical one as well. Because a considerable amount of time usually elapses before a tomographic study

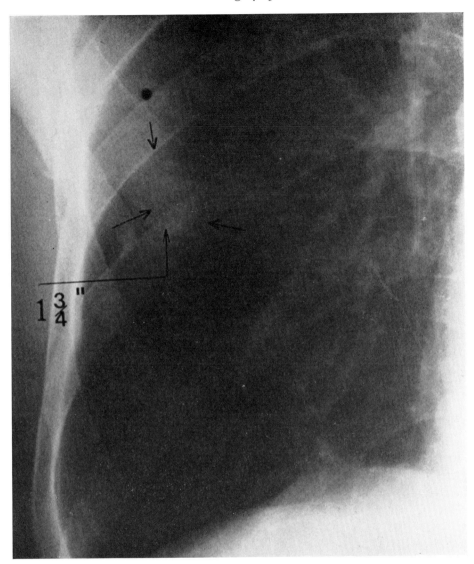

← Figure 180. When measuring the position of the object under examination, the technologist should remember that when the patient lies prone there might be a slight shift in location toward the chest wall. In a lateral chest film, the lesion may be 2.5 inches from the anterior surface; when the patient lies prone, the lesion may be 0.75 to 1 inch from the anterior wall.

is completed, the patient should be kept in as comfortable a position as possible. An appropriate amount of table padding is certainly advisable. If the patient is comfortable he is more likely to cooperate and hold still for longer times. Since the objective plane changes with each adjustment up or down with the fulcrum level, slightly different absorbing rates often occur, producing variations in radiographic density from one film to the

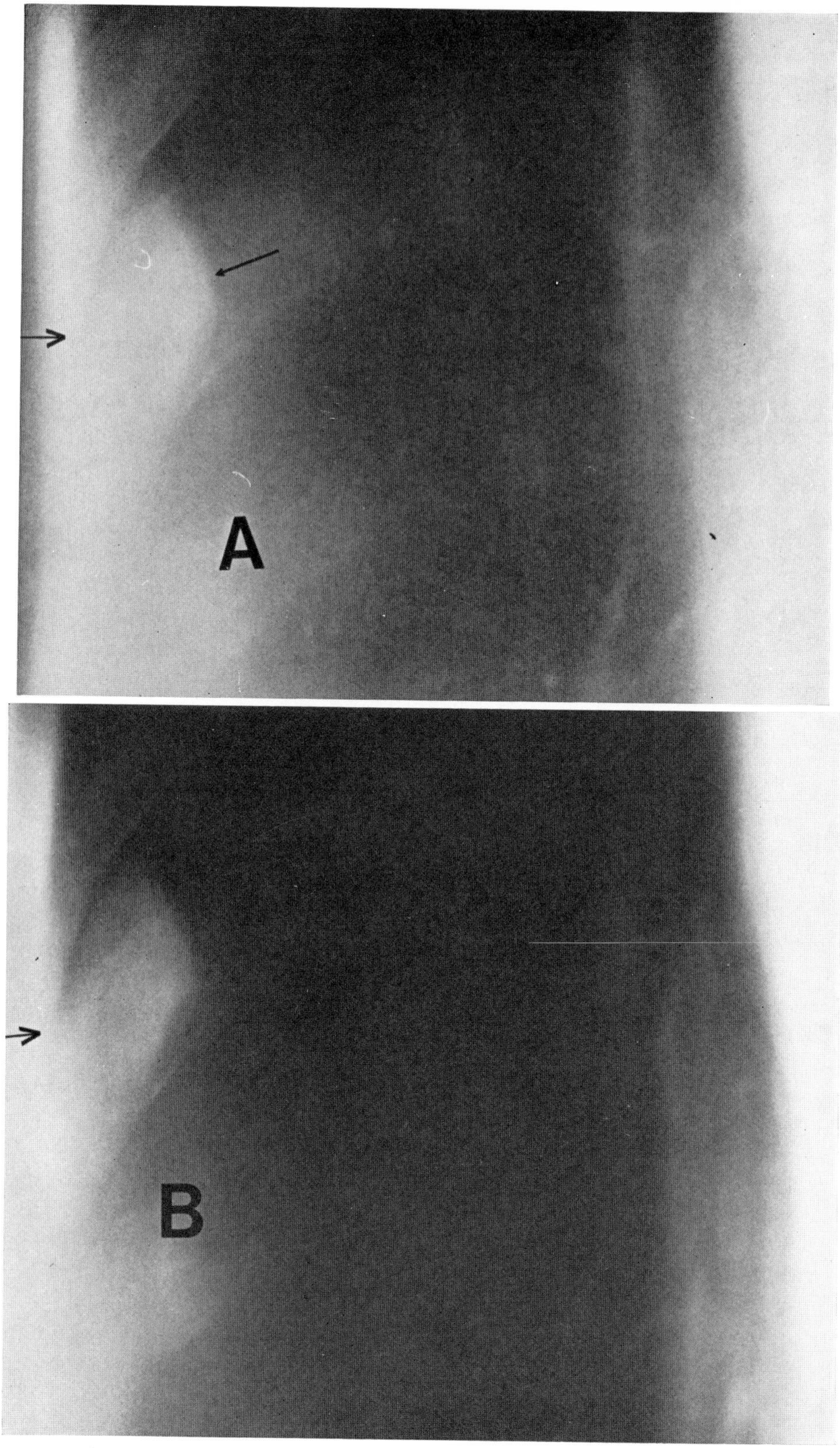
A
B

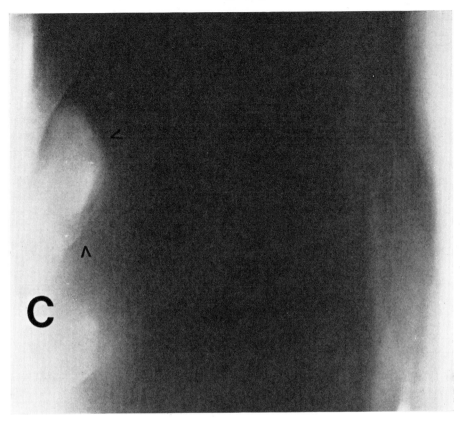

← Figure 181. Variations in density are inevitable when changing fulcrum levels, especially when tomographing areas with high subject contrast.

next. Figure 181 shows this situation. There is nothing that should be done to compensate for this as long as the technologist is reasonably sure that the x-ray equipment is producing the proper amount of exposure each time.

Establishing Exposures for Tomography

Although it is often said that an increase in exposure of 50 percent is required over what was used for a routine film, such adjustments from conventional techniques to tomography actually vary depending on the arc used. A zonogram, for example, will require less exposure when compared to the same body part using a 30 or 40° arc (see Fig. 182).

Types of Linkages

Earlier in the chapter excursion patterns were discussed briefly. It is of some importance that we look into these in more detail now. There are three basic types of linkage systems as noted in Figure 183. (Please

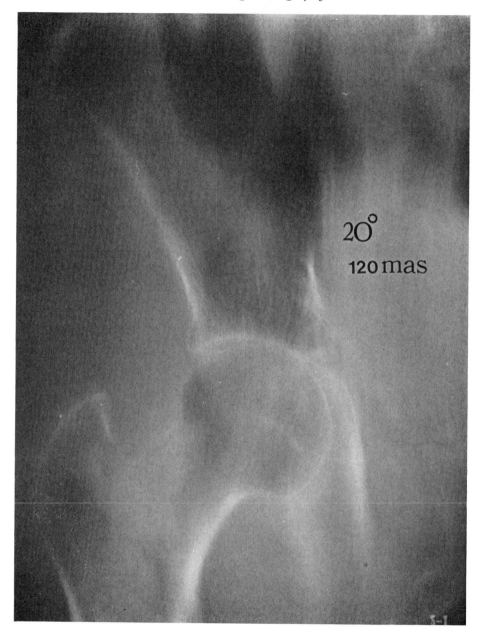

Figure 182A.

Figure 182. Because of the many variables involved, no categorical technique compensations for various arcs can be specified. However, the exposure values used here can be used as a guide.

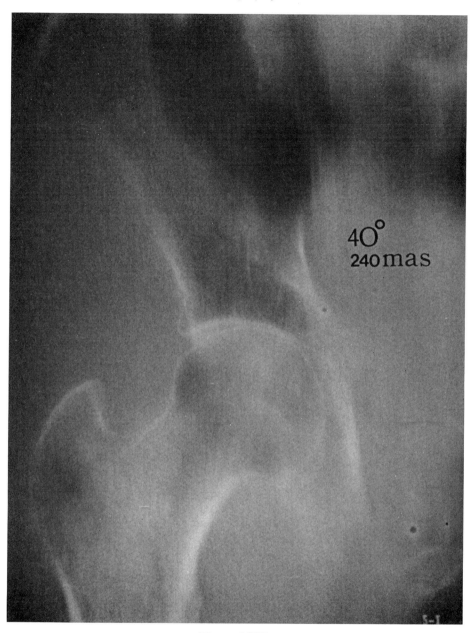

Figure 182B.

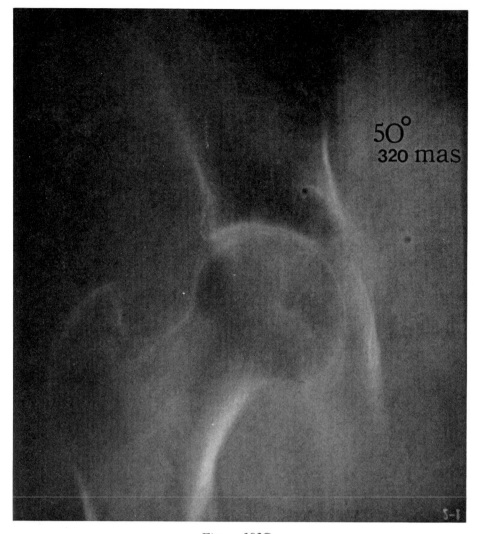

Figure 182C.

note that the ratio between (a), (b), and (c) is important.) Linkage is a term that refers to the method of mechanical connections between the tube and the film. Very often the type of linkage used depends on the manufacturer, and any of these can be used for either linear or pleuri-directional motions. If the tube and film move parallel to each other, we have a line-to-line type of linkage. If the tube moves in an arc but the film moves on a horizontal plane, we have an arc-to-line linkage, and if both the tube and film arc, an arc-to-arc linkage is being used.

The linkage is important to tomographic quality because it influences the sharpness of the objective plane. This one factor, when compared to

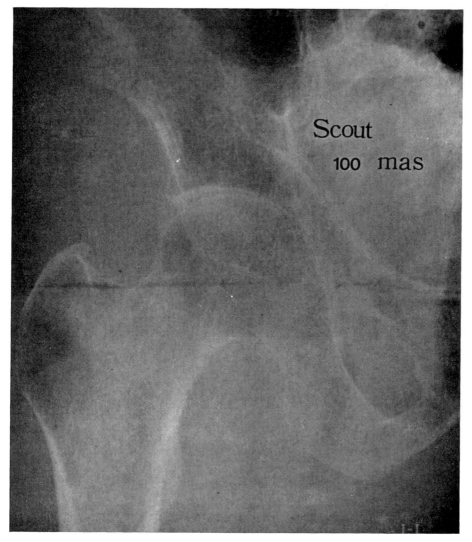

Figure 182D.

the thickness of the cut, the use of book cassettes, and the use of multi-directional patterns, has relatively little effect on the quality of the tomo-graphic image. In general, the arc-to-arc linkage is considered to be the best of the three. The reason for this is that when the tube and film are in motion during the exposure the relationship between the object and the tube and the object and the film with regard to distance is constant. With arc-to-line and the line-to-line types, the object film distance changes somewhat during the exposure and this causes a reduction in the sharp-ness of the objective plane.

LINKAGE FOR LINEAR TOMOGRAPHY

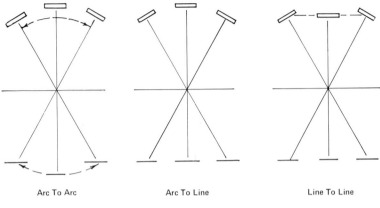

Arc To Arc   Arc To Line   Line To Line

Figure 183.

Pluridirectional Tomography

An important disadvantage regarding (linear) unidirectional tomography has been noted. As tomograms became more popular, there was strong interest in reducing the "smearing" that was common with the simpler linear mechanisms. With linear tomography the smearing (ghost shadows) cannot be avoided. However, with a more complex excursion pattern of the x-ray tube during the exposure these ghost shadows can be virtually eliminated. Figure 176 shows two radiographs that were exposed under the same conditions except one was exposed with a pluridirectional tomographic unit and the other with a linear unit. When you view these radiographs you may come to the conclusion that unless the tube moves in such a way that all structures in the objective plane are transversed ghost shadows will not be eliminated from the tomographic image. As a result, manufacturers began experimenting with these more complex designs and today they are used extensively throughout the country.

As pluridirectional motions were developed, four basic patterns have emerged (Fig. 172 shows these patterns schematically). As one might guess, the most complex of these provides the greatest opportunity for the tube to transverse all structures thus reducing smear and ghost shadows substantially. Smearing, of course, is a kind of half blur and half sharpness that occurs at the transition points which lie between the objective plane and the areas immediately above and below. In other words, the more abrupt a change there is between the sharpness of the objective plane and the total blurring of structures superior and inferior to the plane, the better the objective plane will be. In addition, the need to position the body part under examination in such a way that the tube will move across its long axis is not necessary for pluridirectional tomography. The primary danger with this type of equipment is excess heat at the anode, and very long exposures.

Balancing Exposure Factors for Tomography

A moving tube and film should not preclude the possibility of obtaining good contrast and density. It is the author's opinion that the KvP should not be increased when going from conventional radiography to tomography. There are some who feel that the kilovoltage should be increased; considering the extra thickness of tissue that must be penetrated when the tube is angled for a 40 or 50° arc, there appears at first to be some justification. However, contrast is extremely important when doing tomographic work since thin cuts greatly reduce subject contrast, and so the technique factors should be adjusted so that they produce as much subject contrast as possible. With this in mind, it would be more realistic from a technical point of view to keep the KvP as low as possible and adjust for the density with MaS. This would be especially true with very thin cuts. Figure 184 shows two tomographic images that were made at 10° and 50°, each demonstrating a different radiographic contrast. You will note that the 50° arc cut being thinner has a notable decrease in radiographic contrast.

The Selection of Exposure Angle (Arc)

Figure 185 shows some commonly used arc settings and approximate cut thicknesses they produce, but it should be pointed out that these values may vary slightly between different manufacturers' equipment. There has been no mention, so far, regarding matching the thickness of cut used with the increment of cuts for the tomographic study. Suppose a rather diffuse and moderately large structure was noted in the patient's chest and, as a result, tomograms were ordered. With this situation, it may be important to evaluate the presence of small calcium deposits in the structure as well as the general appearance of the structure itself. If the structure measured 4 cm in size and the technologist made a series of cuts using 1 cm increments, it should also be kept clearly in mind that, if the thickness of the cuts is not matched with the increments from one level to the next, it is possible that some of the structure being examined will not be radiographed at all. Figure 186 shows what can happen if the thickness of the cut obtained is not appropriate or matched with the increments that were used. In short, either the body part will be cut too "fat", or in the case of making thin cuts, with large fulcrum increments, some of the structures will be missed altogether.

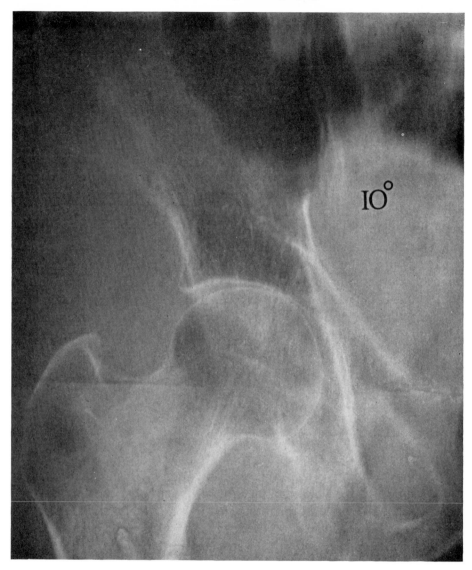

In summary, tomography is a very valuable tool which can be used to improve visualization of structures that are superimposed by other body parts to an extent where they cannot be adequately examined using conventional radiography. The technique utilizes a fulcrum (or pivot point) which provides a level where no tube or film motion is evident. The fulcrum establishes what is known as an objective plane. All structures lying in this plane will be seen in the radiographic image with sufficient sharpness for a radiological diagnosis. The level of the objective plane is adjustable and can be raised or lowered to any point in the body depending on

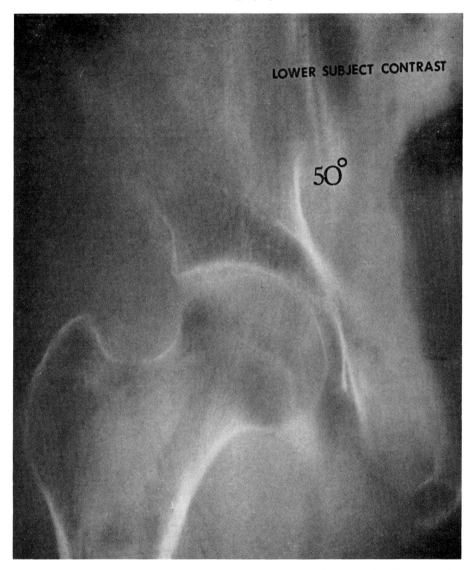

LOWER SUBJECT CONTRAST

50°

← Figure 184. Radiographic contrast decreases as the thickness of the objective plane decreases, because as thinner "slices" of the body are obtained there are fewer objects present to absorb the x-ray beam.

the wishes of the technologist and radiologist. The thickness of the objective plane is dependent on the arc or amplitude, which in turn determines the distance the tube travels *during the exposure*. The greater the exposure arc or amplitude, the greater the distance travelled during the exposure; a thicker cut will result.

There are many types of excursion patterns available ranging from

EXPOSURE ARC	THICKNESS OF CUT
(Degrees)	(mm)
10	6.5
20	3.2
30	2.12
40	1.52
50	1.19

Figure 185. The actual thickness obtained with a given amplitude may vary slightly between units of different tomographic manufacturers. Thickness of cut is a function of the exposure arc and not the complexity of the tube motion.

the simplest rectilinear to the most complex pluridirectional patterns. The major advantage of the more complex types of tube and film motions is that they can reduce the smearing (also called phantom images) of the tomographic image which, of course, increases diagnostic value substantially. An additional increase in exposure is required for tomography over conventional films, but generally these changes should be made by adjusting the MaS and keeping the kilovoltage as low as possible to improve or at least maintain subject contrast. Almost always the exposure must be increased when going from conventional radiography to tomography, but this should be compensated for by increases in MaS. The degree of exposure adjustment necessary for tomography depends on the arc that is to be used. As the exposure arc increases, more tissue is radiated and more exposure will be necessary to produce satisfactory density.

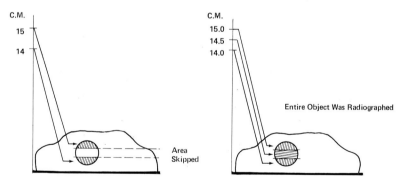

Figure 186. If this concept is not taken into consideration, an important area of an object could be missed unknowingly.

CHAPTER ELEVEN

CONVERSION FACTORS IN RADIOGRAPHY

IN THE FINAL CHAPTER of this text we will discuss the all-important matter of how to review or critique a film for technical quality. As you will see, there are a number of variations possible that can be made by the technologist to correct a technically inadequate radiograph. However, we must first learn how to make adjustments using the four common prime exposure factors and recognize what practical effect these adjustments have on the final radiographic image.

Suppose, for example, a film you have taken is too light because of inadequate penetration. First, we must know or be able to predict how the image will change if we increase the exposure by 5, 10, or 15 kilovolts. In other words, we must know how to increase the KvP so a third repeat exposure and all of the related work in setting up for it will not be necessary. If the lack of sufficient density in our imaginary radiograph is because of insufficient MaS, we must know how much additional MaS is needed to produce the desired effect. In brief, conversion factors and technical adjustments should be made only after we have made a technical diagnosis of the poorly exposed radiographic image.

The second use for conversion factors comes when the technologist is presented with a situation that will not allow the use of the technique posted. Under these conditions, it would be necessary to convert or change the posted exposure factors that are ordinarily used to something that is more compatible to the immediate situation. Experience plays an important role here and, as you watch other technologists improvise and convert their exposure factors for various technical situations, it might be well to ask for a brief explanation at an opportune moment so you can benefit from their experience and expertise.

Any number of such situations may arise, but we will begin with some of the more basic. The first problem might well involve a very sick patient who is not coherent and thus not able to follow breathing instructions adequately. The posted technique for the particular exposure to be made is 200 Ma, 2.5 sec, and 72 KvP. The patient is moving about on the table and so it is clear the exposure time will have to be reduced to

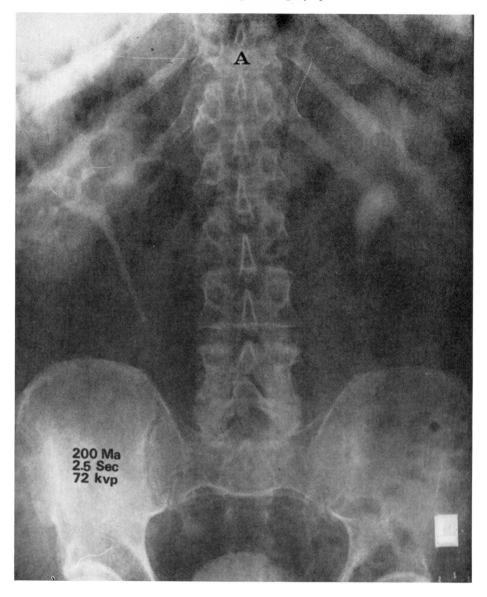

minimize patient motion. Through experience, the technologist who will be responsible for the case knows that any exposure much more than one-half of a second would probably cause too much blurring from patient motion. A situation now exists where the posted technique must be converted to one that will be compatible and will better accommodate the situation at hand. In this example, we will assume the x-ray control panel cannot be used beyond 400 Ma. In Chapter Five we discussed the concept of Ma and time reciprocity, and with this in mind we can proceed with some possible solutions for the problem.

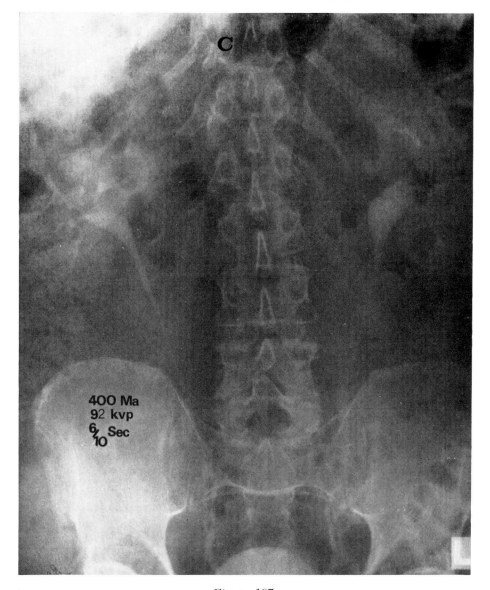

← Figure 187.

You will recall the technique chart was for 200 Ma, however, that will have to be changed to 400 Ma. This allows us to reduce the exposure time from 2.5 sec to 1.25 sec, however, it is feared that this will still be too long an exposure time. Decreasing the focal film distance will certainly increase radiographic density; however, it will also increase magnification and the penumbra (which would not be to our advantage). Kilovoltage can increase radiographic density without producing any negative effect on sharpness or magnification. With this in mind, we will increase the kilovoltage by 12 and this will permit us to lower the exposure time to 0.6 sec. Thus, our new technique to accommodate this situation is 400 Ma, 0.6 sec, at 92 KvP. Figure 187 shows two radiographs, one exposed using the posted technique showing excessive blurring, and the other exposed with the converted technique. There might be other possibilities for finding an acceptable conversion for this situation, but this seems to be the most appropriate.

Another problem might be to try to increase the visibility of detail by producing more contrast in the image. The study is an IVC examination and we want to make the bile ducts as visible as possible radiographically. An experienced technologist would be able to mentally review a list of the items that would potentially improve radiographic contrast. The posted exposure, in this case, is 200 Ma, 0.5 sec, 90 KvP, and the patient's abdomen measures 25 cm A.P. The concept of producing good radiographic contrast was discussed thoroughly. The technical constraints are that the control panel does not go beyond 400 Ma and it is felt that the patient's breathing would become a problem if the exposure time is increased to over one second. In this situation, the reciprocity law by itself would not be of any benefit. The basic problem here is that radiographic contrast is poor. First, coning will be checked and made as tight as possible to reduce the number of excess scatter interactions. Since KvP is so important in determining subject contrast, it is felt that it should be lowered to 70 KvP to produce more differential absorption and less Compton interactions which produce large quantities of scatter. If the Kv is lowered to 70, the resulting radiograph would be too light so we must do something to build up the density lost by reducing the kilovoltage. The first step will be to increase the Ma to 400 (times two), and the Kv will be reduced to 80. If we increase the exposure time to 1 sec (times two) the Kv can be lowered to 70. The converted technique then is 400 Ma, 1 sec, at 70 KvP. It should be mentioned, also, that compression can be used in such a situation, if possible medically, to help increase radiographic density. In fact, depending on whether the patient is really flabby, sufficient compression might allow a further reduction of KvP to approximately 66 without danger of insufficient radiographic density. One could also use a very fast pair of screens (rare earth) if available which would allow a further reduction of exposure time to 0.5 sec (beware of quantum mottle).

Portable and operating room work often requires a good deal of technical imagination and ingenuity. Orthopedic work can be especially trying and portable grid work can be very demanding. Let us discuss a circumstance where a cross bed lateral hip must be performed to check for postoperative alignment of the broken fragment. The patient, however, was in bed in a way that caused increased object film distance, resulting in a

$\rightarrow$

Figure 188. A series of radiographs exposed with longer times. It would be very helpful for the technologist, when calculating exposures for repeat films, to note the increments of times and the respective density values obtained.

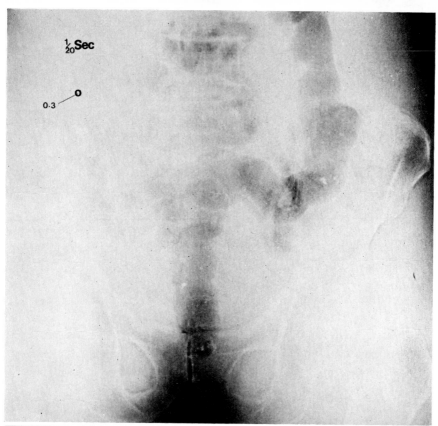

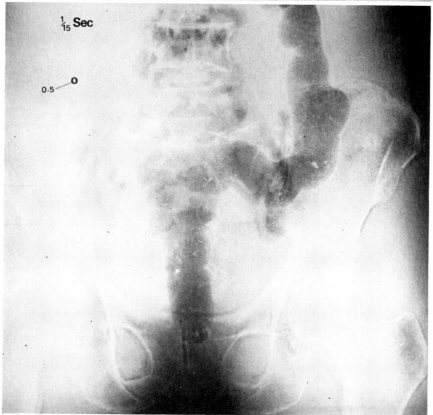

Figures 188A and B.

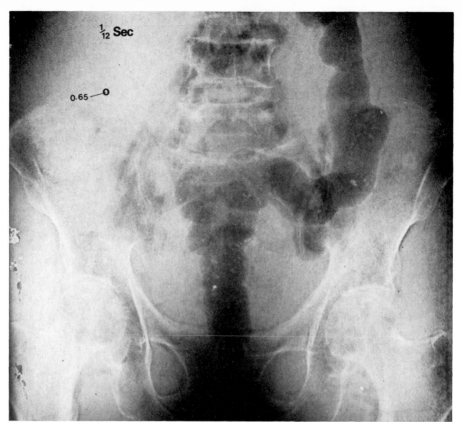

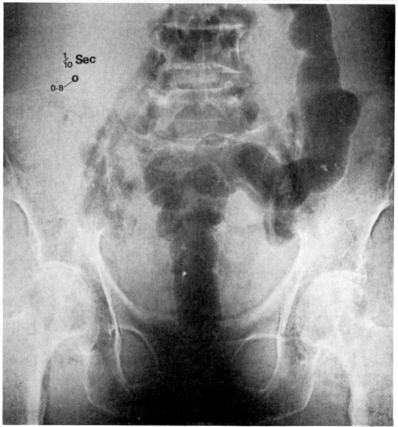

Figures 188C and D.

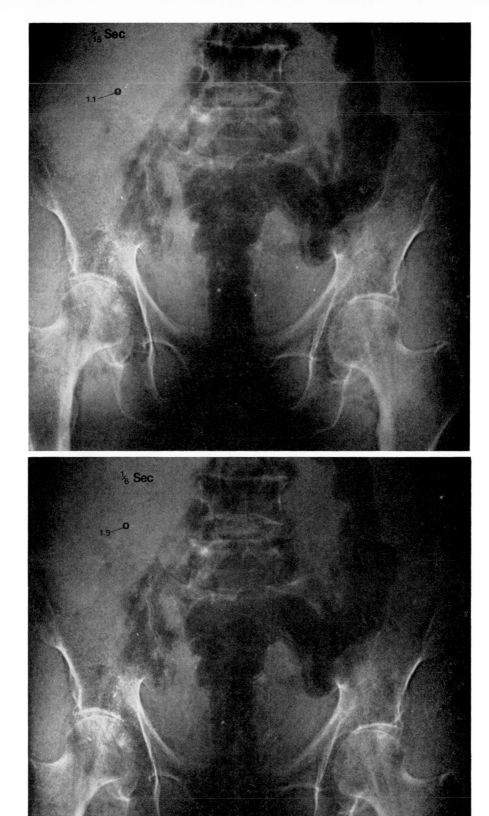

Figures 188E and F.

considerable amount of penumbra and magnification. You will recall that magnification greatly increases the effect of penumbra by the divergent rays emitted from the target. Since, in this case, object film distance cannot be reduced for the exposure, its effect on the radiographic image can be reduced substantially by increasing the F.F.D. The object film distance was, in fact, 6 inches and the portable unit was originally set for 200 MaS at 80 KvP at 40 inches focal film distance. The 6-inch object film distance could be effectively compromised by using 60-inch focal film distance, but this would cause, of course, a reduction in radiographic density and the technologist must convert his original exposure factors accordingly. In this situation, the portable unit has no Ma station above 200. Recalling the inverse square law, if the focal film distance is increased by 50 percent, the radiographic density will be reduced to one half of what it was originally. Since the Ma and time factors must be held constant in this particular situation, it is necessary to increase the kilovoltage to 94, which would make our converted technique 200 MaS, 60 inches F.F.D., at 92 KvP.

Another requisition may come along involving the use of a grid where

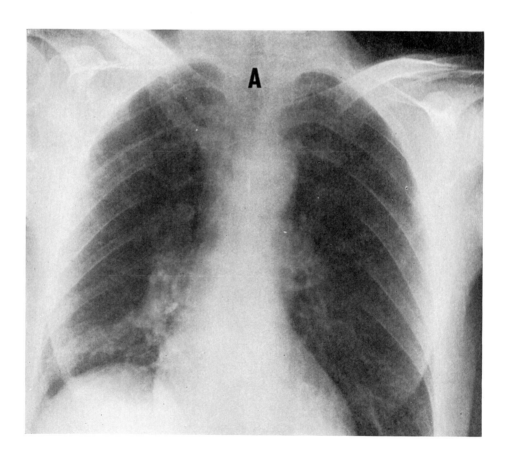

it was not used previously. A chest film, for example, was made on a very heavy patient nongrid and had too much fog caused by excessive secondary scatter radiation. The technologist chose a 5:1 grid for the second exposure to reduce the number of scatter rays reaching the film. The original exposure was 5 MaS at 80 KvP and since the grid will absorb much scatter, the radiographic density will be greatly reduced. The new technique using a 5:1 grid was increased subsequently to 16 MaS at 80 KvP. Figure 189 shows these two radiographs for comparison.

Another situation may arise when doing extremities using direct exposure technique where the patient cannot hold still for the long exposures needed for nonscreen radiography. The technologist chooses to use a cassette with par speed screens, so the original exposure must be reduced drastically to compensate for the intensification factor of the screens. The original technique (Fig. 190B) was 50 KvP, 100 Ma, at 3 sec and was converted to 100 Ma, $\frac{1}{15}$ sec, at 50 KvP (Fig. 190A).

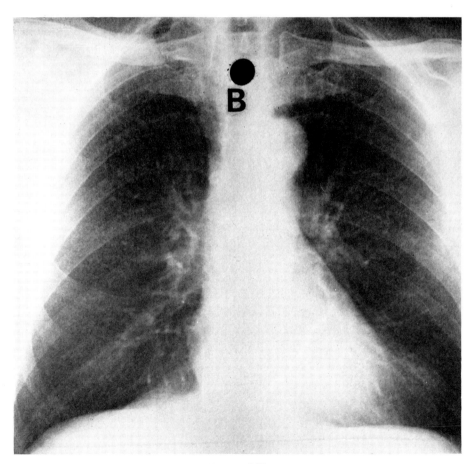

←   Figure 189.

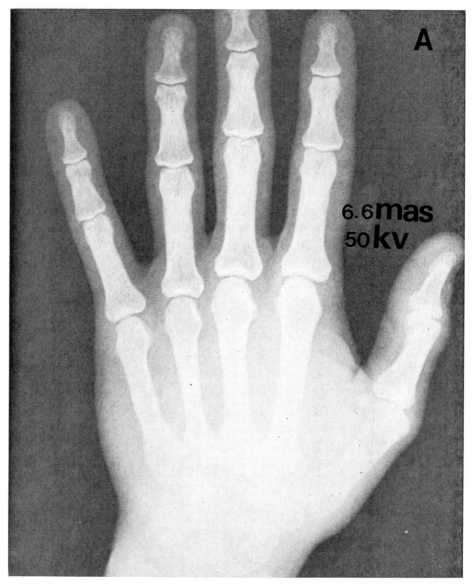

When additional contrast is required as a result of too much scatter fog reaching the film, one may always use a grid cassette or a stationary grid taped to a cassette, which is then placed in the bucky tray. If a second grid is used in this way to supplement the one already used in the bucky tray, additional absorption of the remnant radiation is obvious. To keep from overloading the tube one may often successfully use a very high speed, rare earth screen. It is worth noting here that when two grids are used in this way one can easily afford to increase KvP substantially without fear of scatter fog detracting from radiographic quality.

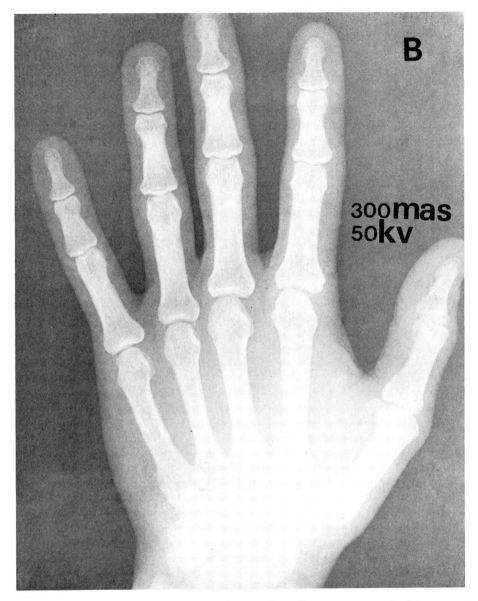

Figure 190. The nonscreen (*B*, exposed in cardboard) exposure required is approximately forty times more than the screen (*A*, par speed screen) exposure.

As you will recall, high KvP at low MaS exposures is also considerably less damaging to the tube than vice versa.

CONVERSION FACTORS

There is no question that the converted techniques noted above could have been arrived at through lucky guesses; however, a more reliable method of making these technical changes would result from using or at least becoming familiar with various conversion factors that will be presented in this chapter. It is appropriate, at this point, to remind the student that a technologist is often measured by the consistency with which he produces good radiographic examinations. To produce an occasional "pretty" or exceptional film is certainly to one's credit, but it is also simply a stroke of fortunate luck and does not necessarily indicate a talented technologist.

Very often technologists have a tendency to emphasize a few of these rare "Roentgen Rembrandts" and forget the majority of the marginal cases they have produced throughout a given week or month. The author has worked with many talented technologists who have developed their abilities wisely, and also those who have learned to become good technologists through practice and effort. In any case, the most valued technologist is the one who can produce good radiographs consistently. Fortunately, there are reliable methods that can be used to calculate new conversion factors mentally during the examination if necessary. Although there are many such conversion formulas to know depending on the situation, only a few are used with any degree of regularity. If one becomes familiar with these few it will prove very beneficial to both the technologist and the patient. To make the problem of conversions more manageable the author will introduce the concept of the conversion factor or "C" factor. This can be used effectively for practically any radiographic situation similar to those noted above. The reader will take note that KvP conversions (see Table II) are not written merely in increments of 10. Because of the effect exposure latitude has with decreasing and increasing changes in KvP, it is misleading and incorrect for the technologist to do so because it often results in an incorrect choice of exposure factors.

Increasing the KvP, for example, will give much different results depending on the KvP level of the original film. An alternate method is to think in terms of increasing or decreasing the exposure by increments of 15 or 7 percent (see Fig. 191). In Table III, you will note formulas that can be used to find the new time or Ma when the other has been changed. Other conversion tables and formulas have been included to aid in finding the correct conversion factors.

Two final points must be made before concluding this chapter. First the contrast of the film has a very important role in calculating conversion factors. You will find that high contrast film will yield more dramatic radiographic changes in the image when the same conversion factor is used. For example, if we used a high contrast film and a low contrast film and had an original technique of 15 MaS at 70 Kv, then increased the

TABLE II
KvP — DENSITY CALCULATIONS

New KvP→	Density +50% Column A	Density +100% Column B	Density −25% Column C	Density −50% Column D
Initial KvP	(Plus 7%)	(Plus 15%)	(Minus 7%)	(Minus 15%)
50 :	53	57	46	42
52 :	55	59	48	44
54 :	57	62	50	45
56 :	59	64	52	47
58 :	62	66	53	49
60 :	64	69	55	51
62 :	66	71	57	52
64 :	68	73	59	54
66 :	70	75	61	56
68 :	72	78	63	57
70 :	74	80	65	59
72 :	77	82	66	61
74 :	79	85	68	62
76 :	81	87	70	64
78 :	83	89	72	66
80 :	85	92	74	68
82 :	87	94	76	69
84 :	89	96	78	71
86 :	92	98	79	73
88 :	94	101	81	74
90 :	96	103	83	76
92 :	98	105	85	78
94 :	100	108	87	79
96 :	102	110	89	81
98 :	104	112	91	83
100 :	107	115	93	85
102 :	109	117	94	86
104 :	111	119	96	88
106 :	113	121	98	90
108 :	115	124	100	91
110 :	117	126	102	93
112 :	119	128	104	95
114 :	121	131	106	96
116 :	124	133	107	98
118 :	126	135	109	100
120 :	128	138	111	102
122 :	130	140	113	103
124 :	132	142	115	105
126 :	134	144	117	107
128 :	136	147	119	108
130 :	139	149	120	110

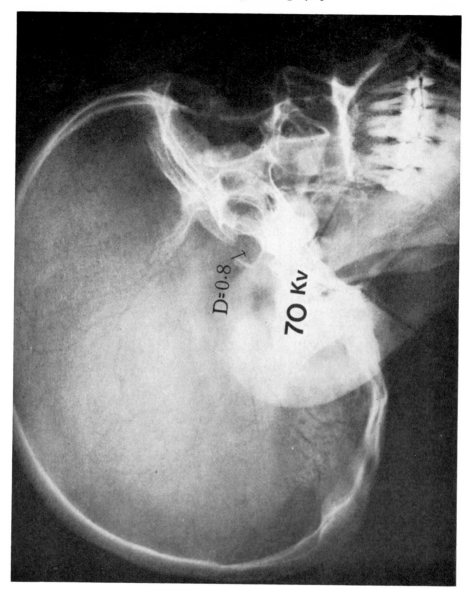

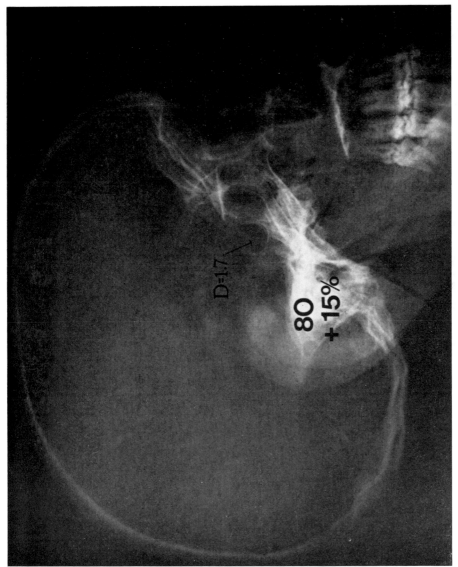

Figure 191. These radiographs show the effect in density with a 15 percent increase in KvP. If more subtle changes in density are required, the author's experience is that an 8 percent increase in KvP will prove adequate.

TABLE III

CONVERSION TABLES

It must be kept in mind that the conversion factors below were established under controlled conditions. Because of the tremendous number of variables involving film type, processing conditions, type of screens, various KvP levels, filtrations, generator calibrations, and the variety of factors affecting body habitus, it is simply impossible to have categorical conversion factors that will work equally well under all situations. However, because medical x-ray film has wide latitude characteristics, the conversion factors noted below will provide diagnostic radiographic images.

I. How to find the exposure time and Ma from a given MaS value.

A. $$\frac{MaS}{The\ Ma\ Desired} = Exposure\ Time$$

PROBLEM: If MaS is given as 71, what would the time be if 200 Ma is desired?

$$\frac{71\ MaS}{200\ Ma} = \frac{35}{100} = \frac{7}{20}\ sec$$

Please note that if 7/20 is not on the timer selector, the available time can be estimated by using the following logic: Since 10/20 equals 1/2 and 5/20 equals 1/4, 7/20 would be close to the midpoint of 1/4 and 1/2 so the nearest time to this point can be used.

B. $$\frac{MaS}{The\ Time\ Desired} = Milliamperage$$

PROBLEM: If 71 MaS is given, what would the Ma be at a desired time of 1/2 second?

$$\frac{71\ MaS}{1/2\ sec} = 140\ Ma$$

Because of the many time stations available, it is usually better to choose the desired Ma and calculate for the exposure time.

II. How to find the new Ma when the exposure time has been changed.

$$\frac{Original\ Ma \times Original\ Time}{New\ Time} = New\ Ma$$

PROBLEM: Originally, the exposure was made at 100 Ma at 1/4 sec. What would the new Ma be if the time is changed to 1/20 sec?

$$\frac{100 \times 1/4}{1/20} \times \frac{25}{.05} \times 500\ Ma$$

III. How to find the new exposure time when the Ma has been changed.

$$\frac{Original\ Ma \times Original\ Time}{New\ Ma} = New\ Time$$

PROBLEM: If the initial exposure is made at 500 Ma at 1/2 sec, what would the time be at an exposure of 200 Ma?

$$\frac{500 \times 1/2}{200} = 1.25\ sec$$

IV. How to find the new Ma or MaS or time when the distance is changed.

$$\frac{Original\ MaS \times (New\ F.F.D.)^2}{(Original\ F.F.D.)^2} = New\ MaS$$

TABLE III—*Continued*

CONVERSION TABLES

Note that time, Ma, or MaS values can be interchanged whenever these calculations are made.

PROBLEM: If the exposure is 5 MaS at a distance of thirty inches, what would the exposure be at a distance of forty inches?

$$\frac{5 \times 40^2}{30^2} = \frac{8000}{900} = 9 \text{ MaS}$$

V.   How to find the new exposure when only a slight change in density is needed.

To increase: Original MaS × 1.25 = New MaS
               Original KvP × 1.08 = New KvP

To decrease: Original MaS × 0.75 = New MaS
               Original KvP × 0.93 = New KvP

VI.   How to change the radiographic density.

Original MaS × 1.5 =   50% increase
Original MaS × 2.0 = 100% increase
Original MaS × 3.0 = 150% increase
Original MaS × 0.75 = 25% decrease
Original MaS × 0.50 = 50% decrease
Original MaS × 0.25 = 75% decrease

VII.   How to change the radiographic density (also see Figure 191 and Table II).

Original KvP × 1.08 =   50% increase
Original KvP × 1.15 = 100% increase
Original KvP × 1.23 = 150% increase
Original KvP × .93 = 25% decrease
Original KvP × .85 = 50% decrease
Original KvP × .78 = 75% decrease

VIII.   How to find the new MaS when coning is sharply increased (from open field to a tight spot).

Original MaS × 1.35 = New MaS
Original KvP × 1.08 = New KvP

Note that these conversions will vary depending on the amount of S/S radiation present in the original exposure.

IX.   Alternate method for calculating new time, MaS, or Ma when the distance is changed·

New F.F.D.² ÷ Original F.F.D.² × Original MaS = New MaS

X.   How to make quick estimates when focal film distance is altered.

25% increase, from 40 to 50 inches: Original MaS × 1.5 = New MaS
                                        Original KvP × 1.08 = New KvP

50% increase, from 40 to 60 inches: Original MaS × 2.25 = New MaS
                                        Original KvP × 1.23 = New KvP

100% increase, from 40 to 80 inches: Original MaS × 4 = New MaS
                                        Original KvP × 1.3 = New KvP

10% decrease, from 40 to 36 inches: Original MaS × 0.8 = New MaS
                                        Original KvP × 0.94 = New KvP

25% decrease, from 40 to 30 inches: Original MaS × 0.55 = New MaS
                                        Original KvP × 0.85 = New KvP

50% decrease, from 40 to 20 inches: Original MaS × 0.25 = New MaS
                                        Original KvP × 0.72 = New KvP

XI.   How to find the new MaS, time, or Ma when changing screens (at 65 KvP).

Direct exposure to detail speed: Original MaS × 0.043 = New MaS

Direct exposure to medium speed: Original MaS × 0.022 = New MaS

TABLE III—*Continued*

CONVERSION TABLES

Direct exposure to fast speed: Original MaS × 0.011 = New MaS

Direct exposure to rare earth: Original MaS × 0.006 = New MaS

Detail speed to nonscreen: Original MaS × 23   = New MaS

Medium speed to nonscreen: Original MaS × 46   = New MaS

Fast speed to nonscreen: Original MaS × 87   = New MaS

Rare earth to nonscreen: Original MaS × 170   = New MaS

Please note that most screens are made with speed factors in multiples of 2: A fast speed screen is two times faster than medium, so the exposure must be decreased to one-half of the original; a medium speed screen is two times faster than detail speed, so the exposure must be reduced to one-half of the original value.

XII.   How to change grids (the conversion factors will vary slightly depending on the KvP, part thickness, density, and general body habitus).

At 75 KvP:

From no grid to 5:1 grid: Original MaS × 1.5   = New MaS

From no grid to 6:1 grid: Original MaS × 2.0   = New MaS

From no grid to 8:1 grid: Original MaS × 3.0   = New MaS

From no grid to 12:1 grid: Original MaS × 3.5   = New MaS

From 5:1 grid to 6:1 grid: Original MaS × 1.5   = New MaS
                                Original KvP × 1.08 = New KvP

From 5:1 grid to 8:1 grid: Original MaS × 2.0   = New MaS
                                Original KvP × 1.15 = New KvP

From 5:1 grid to 12:1 grid: Original MaS × 2.33 = New Mas
                                Original KvP × 1.30 = New KvP

From 6:1 grid to 8:1 grid: Original MaS × 1.5   = New MaS
                                Original KvP × 1.08 = New KvP

From 6:1 grid to 12:1 grid: Original MaS × 1.75 = New MaS
                                Original KvP × 1.11 = New KvP

From 8:1 grid to 12:1 grid: Original MaS × 1.5   = New MaS
                                Original KvP × 1.09 = New KvP

From 12:1 grid to 8:1 grid: Original MaS × 0.75 = New MaS
                                Original KvP × 0.95 = New KvP

From 12:1 grid to 6:1 grid: Original MaS × 0.55 = New MaS
                                Original KvP × 0.88 = New KvP

From 12:1 grid to 5:1 grid: Original MaS × 0.43 = New MaS
                                Original KvP × 0.75 = New KvP

From 8:1 grid to 6:1 grid: Original MaS × 0.66 = New MaS
                                Original KvP × 0.93 = New KvP

From 8:1 grid to 5:1 grid: Original MaS × 0.5   = New MaS
                                Original KvP × 0.85 = New KvP

From 6:1 grid to 5:1 grid: Original MaS × 0.75 = New MaS
                                Original KvP × 0.95 = New KvP

exposure by 50 percent, the high contrast film would show a greater effect
on the image than would the low contrast film, as indicated:

Exposure	Radiographic Density	
	High Contrast Film	Low Contrast Film
15 MaS	0.8	0.8
22.5 MaS	1.4	1.1

The second point that must be made regarding the effect a conversion
factor has on the radiographic image is dependent on where the original
density of the film *lies* on the H & D curve. If all other factors are constant, it is very likely that the same conversion factor will produce a
different effect on the density of the image (see Fig. 192).

When the density of the original film lies close to the toe or shoulder of the
H & D curve, the technologist should be mindful that a slightly greater adjustment in technique for the repeat is usually necessary.

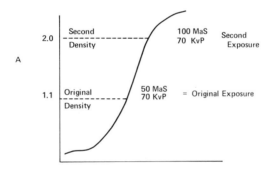

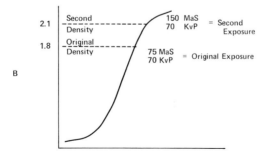

Figure 192. X-ray film is not able to record densities increasing beyond 1.5 in proportion to increasing exposure values. In *A* and *B* the MaS was doubled from the
original density. However, *A* does not produce the same effect in density as *B*. This
is one important reason why it is difficult and misleading to make categorical statements about the effect any one specific conversion factor will have on the radiographic
image.

Experience has taught the author that more often than not technologists are too conservative when estimating how light or dark their original radiograph appears and consequently make too small an adjustment in exposure factors. It is very important for students to learn to make accurate estimates in determining how light or dark the original film is from what is considered to be optimal. Only then can he hope to make consistently accurate technical adjustments for the repeat films. It is also strongly recommended that he learn to express these differences in density in terms of percentages, such as this film is 50 percent darker than it should be or this film is 50 percent lighter than optimal for this exam. Once this information is determined, the exposure may be increased or decreased by 50 percent according to the tables. With this system, the technologist has better control over his finished work, and radiography becomes something more than a mere guessing game. It might be helpful to have a small library of films exposed deliberately with different factors. A densitometer can then be used to get a reading that represents their overall densities. During film critique classes, these films may be presented to train and test abilities in correctly estimating how light or dark the images are from what is thought to be optimal.

CHAPTER TWELVE

FILM CRITIQUE

V ERY SHORTLY after Roentgen's discovery of x-radiation, many physicians began experimenting with this amazing phenomenon for possible applications in the medical field. By the early 1900s the usefulness of x-radiation in helping determine fractured bones had been documented, but as time went on physicians, in cooperation with physicists, began to realize that this new medium could be used for purposes other than the mere visualization of bony fragments and dislocations.

By 1910, the use of x-rays was almost commonplace, and experimentation with other medical applications had, by that time, built to almost a fever pitch. More and more medical facilities had acquired x-ray equipment for the first time, and those facilities that were fortunate enough had additional equipment installed for newly developed uses and research. It was indeed a rare moment in medical history. As the use of x-rays continued to grow, it became clear that physicians who had a special interest in this aspect of medical care had little time available for the more traditional methods of practicing medicine and before too long the A.M.A. recognized the need and the practicality for a new medical specialty known as Roentgenology. The roentgenologist, as he was known in those days, performed all the required procedures necessary to produce a roentgenographic image until the demands in interpreting the plates caused him to seek people to help with the more functionary duties of making the exposure and processing the plates. From these humble beginnings the x-ray technologist has evolved into today's highly trained, sophisticated technologist who has continued to grow with the changing demands of the medical profession. Not only has the diagnostic application of x-ray technology continued to grow but many subspecialties have evolved as well; this has, in turn, increased the demands of their technical knowledge even further.

In the realm of modern radiographic technology, the technologist is playing a more dominant role than he had in the past. Today many radiology residents receive abbreviated theory and little or no practical training regarding the writing of technique charts and the actual application of such accessory equipment as intensifying screens, grids, and processing film.

More and more, the responsibility for the truly technical aspects of radiology are being delegated to technologists. Most radiological technologists welcome this responsibility because it offers more opportunity to grow as professionals and to develop their departments to produce a higher quality radiographic study and interpretation by the radiologist.

Today the radiologist and the technologist work as a team to achieve the end result of producing a high quality radiographic diagnosis for the patients referred to them by private physicians. With this responsibility, cooperation, and recognition of the technologist as a thoroughly trained radiation worker, it is important for us to function in such a way as to not only maintain this growth but further develop this trust by conscientiously learning the basic concepts of how and, equally important, why certain radiographic problems manifest themselves and how to make the appropriate corrections when necessary. This is, above all else, the fundamental purpose and responsibility of today's radiologic technologist. With this idea firmly fixed in our minds, we will begin a review of the various characteristics we should want to produce in the radiographic image.

The immediate task at hand will be to review some of the important terms that will directly pertain to the matter in this chapter. The first of these is density, a general term used to describe the blackness of a radiograph or a specific area. Density is measured with a device known as a densitometer, which measures the tones of radiographic density in quantitative terms such as 1.5^D. The diagnostic tone range for most studies lies between $.25^D$ and 2.0^D.

Radiographic contrast is the difference between two or more tones of density in a radiographic image. The optimal amount of contrast and density desired in an image is purely subjective and cannot be given a specific value. Contrast *scale* refers to the tonal differences of a series of densities ranging from the darkest to the lightest tone. You will recall that if there is an abrupt difference in the tones (the tonal range from black to white happens very quickly) you are looking at a short (high) scale contrast. If, however, the differences between the various neighboring tones is subtle and one observes total range of these tones from black to white very gradually, you are viewing a long (low) contrast scale. It should be made very clear that for routine studies neither extreme is optimal, but rather something in between is desired. Figure 193 shows samples of these variations in contrast scale.

Definition or sharpness is another concept that must be understood. Blurred structures, of course, cause a loss in diagnostic information and

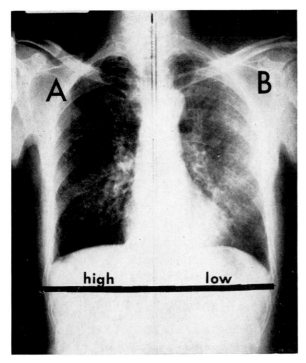

Figure 193. Two films with different contrast characteristics (*A* is a high contrast film, *B* is a low contrast film) were cut to fit into the cassette. One exposure was made, and both halves were processed at the same time to eliminate any variables.

should be avoided. It is not by coincidence that contrast, density, and sharpness were reviewed first. A radiograph, to have optimal detail, must have sufficient contrast to see or differentiate the various structures of the body, it must have enough density or overall accumulation of black metallic silver to present the various body structures, and finally it must possess definition so the structures being viewed are sharply defined or delineated in the image. If the various structures did not have well defined borders, each would "melt" (blur) together making their evaluation or diagnosis impossible. Thus, it is these three characteristics that are considered prerequisites for good radiographic quality.

The terms detail and image quality should be reviewed as well. The remnant x-ray beam is a media that transfers an impression (via variations in intensity) onto the film's emulsion. If all possible conditions are properly set, they will be recorded by the film, and processing will make visible the desired body structures that are to be examined. If, however, something is amiss with either contrast, density, or sharpness, the required reproduction of the body part will not be seen adequately. Detail is the ease with which the viewer can see small structures in the image, and quality is a more general term used to describe the overall diagnostic value of the radiographic image.

VISIBILITY AND DEFINITION OF DETAIL

The radiographic image can be analyzed from two distinct points of view. These two areas are visibility of detail and definition of detail. In order to critique (analyze) a film effectively one must *first* be able to tell the difference between visibility problems and definition problems. It was pointed out earlier in the text that visibility of detail refers to the ability to see the structures under examination. Figure 194 shows two radiographs that have very little visibility of detail. One image possesses very poor contrast and the other image is too dark to make visible the structures or detail that has been impressed into the film's emulsion by the projected image. Visibility of detail then is how well one can see or visualize body parts that *are present* in the emulsion.

The Effect of Contrast on Visibility of Detail

With the understanding that visibility of detail means the ease with which detail can be "seen" in the image, a brief review of all the factors that affect visibility is in order. With this as a starting point, contrast should be considered among the most important. In Figure 193, there is no question as to which radiograph has greater visibility of detail and diagnostic value.

Many factors affect radiographic contrast, and it would be misleading to list them in order of importance because each of the items shown in Figure 195 can cause equally urgent technical problems. It would be helpful, however, to list them in the order of probability of occurrence so when one begins to critique a radiograph with poor contrast an appropriate starting point can be more easily found. Throughout the text, much time was given in describing various causes and remedies of poor radiographic contrast. As a supplement to these discussions it is advisable that Figure 195 be reviewed.

Trying to find the cause of poor contrast can be an extremely difficult problem to isolate because contrast has so many contributing factors. On the other hand, if a radiograph is too dense, usually the technologist need only know how much of a reduction of exposure (MaS) is needed, or, if overpenetration is suspected, the KvP should be reduced to achieve the required results.

The technologist must first realize that contrast is indeed poor, then a technical diagnosis must be made that will help him find the cause of the poor contrast. To do this properly, a basic knowledge of x-ray principles

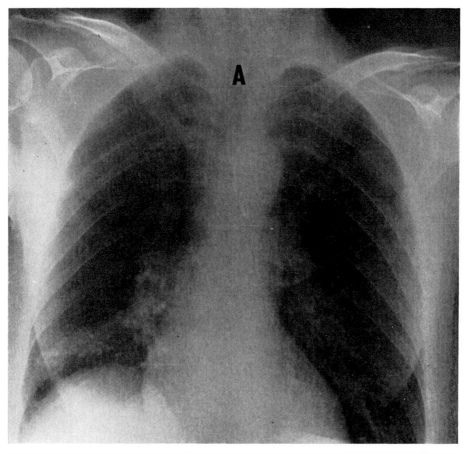

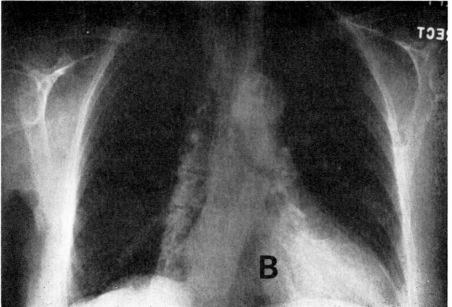

Figure 194. The total diagnostic value of the films is diminished as a result of poor visibility of detail.

MAJOR FACTORS THAT AFFECT RADIOGRAPHIC CONTRAST

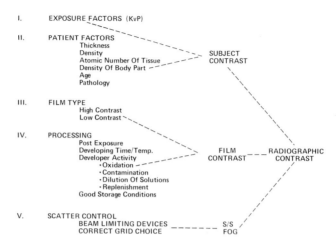

Figure 195.

must be well in hand and a few additional years of experience and practice is certainly helpful. The technologist must train himself to become a good technical diagnostician and to do this effectively. Later in this chapter, radiographs taken during a routine working schedule will be critiqued and compared with the corrected exposure settings. An important point to remember when making corrections for poor radiographic contrast is that frequently there is more than one factor contributing to the undesirable image so that it is necessary to mentally review more than one or two items.

In the case of density, the technical diagnosis and solution to the problem is usually more straightforward than with contrast. It would not be good practice to increase the F.F.D., for example, because of the focused grid and the limitation with the height of the ceiling. Also, changes in focal film distance would affect the sharpness of the radiographic image as well as density. Similarly it would not be appropriate to reduce KvP because of the possible effect on radiographic contrast as well as the possibility of insufficient penetration. More realistically, corrections for density are made by changing the time or the Ma (MaS). In the section covering conversions we saw the effect MaS changes had on density.

There are adjustments that could be made with processing, film, or screens; however, these items should be held as a constant and not used as additional factors to correct exposure problems. Changing developer activity through replenishment or by temperature could lead to more complicated problems. For the purpose of correcting poor contrast or density, one should be keenly aware of the fact that the vast majority of poor quality radiographs are the result of improper exposure factors and not processing, grids, film, or screens.

The following summary of probable causes for poor radiographic quality due to visibility of detail may be helpful.

Artifacts	Dirty screens
	Static
	Fingerprints on the film
	Scratches from the processor
Body habitus	Elderly patient—absorption is poor
	—poor subject contrast
	Pathology
	Obese patient—poor subject contrast
Poor contrast	Excessive S/S reaching the film
	KvP set too high
	Excessive base fog
Density	Incorrect exposure factors
	Chemical fog
	Using wrong film/screen combination
	Improperly positioned grid—light film
Penetration (KvP)	Body too thick or dense for KvP—poor penetration
Processing	Chemical fog
	Under replenishment
	Over replenishment
	Contaminated solutions
	High developing temperature

Sharpness of Detail

Throughout the discussion of visibility of detail it was presumed the body structures have sharply defined borders or edges and these must be seen as such in the radiographic image, but because of contrast or density problems these structures are not seen easily. This concept is illustrated in Figure 196, a photograph of dashes sharply impressed in the page, yet the image of a circle cannot be seen as such in B because the overall density and contrasts do not allow easy visualization of the dashes. Also, we may use the example of trying to visualize a ship sailing in the midst of a heavy fog. The structure of the ship with its sharply defined lines are certainly present yet because of the overall fog its structures are not seen. The problem is not because of poor definition. In radiography the same type of condition exists when a radiographic image is too dense or has too much fog to see the various structures that have been placed in the image by the projected beam.

In the case of sharpness or definition of detail we are concerned with actual delineation and sharpness of the borders of each body structure. Figure 197 shows examples of good sharpness and poor sharpness. This

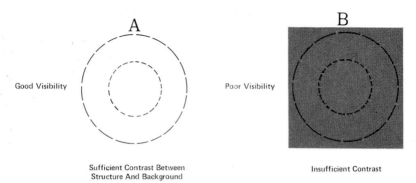

Figure 196. The geometric aspects of the image are optimal. However, they are not visible in film because the density and contrast portion of the technical image is poorly balanced.

factor (sharpness of detail) is controlled by those factors that affect or influence the projected (or geometric) beam, which include intensifying screens. It is the projection (geometry of the photons in the beam) that determine sharpness of detail. The actual detail or information is carried from the patient by the remnant beam and is implanted into the film's emulsion. At that moment the geometric structure (borders) of the image is present, and it is the responsibility of contrast and density to make the various structures optimally visible. In Figure 198 you will be able to see this as you look at the simulated x-ray photons pass through a wire mesh and carry the impression of the structure to the film. This information containing the structural and border lines of the body part under examination is known as the geometric or projected image and is totally responsible for definition of detail.

Thus there are two separate components to every x-ray beam, those related to visibility of detail and those related to definition of detail. When critiquing a radiograph one must first be able to differentiate between the two. Further, one must keep in mind that visibility problems are directly related to radiographic contrast and density and problems related to definition of detail are related to radiographic blurring or distortion.

AN APPROACH TO FILM CRITIQUE

If one would watch a radiologist as he interprets a film and reaches a diagnosis, one would begin to realize that he uses a somewhat fixed regimen. While viewing a PA chest examination, for example, he may first look at the bones of the right side then the left and go on in each progressive step until he has seen the entire film.

$\rightarrow$

Figure 197. *A* reveals acceptable sharpness of the structures in the body. In *B* the borders of the body parts are poorly defined. This unsharpness at first may seem minimal, but much important information could be lost as a result.

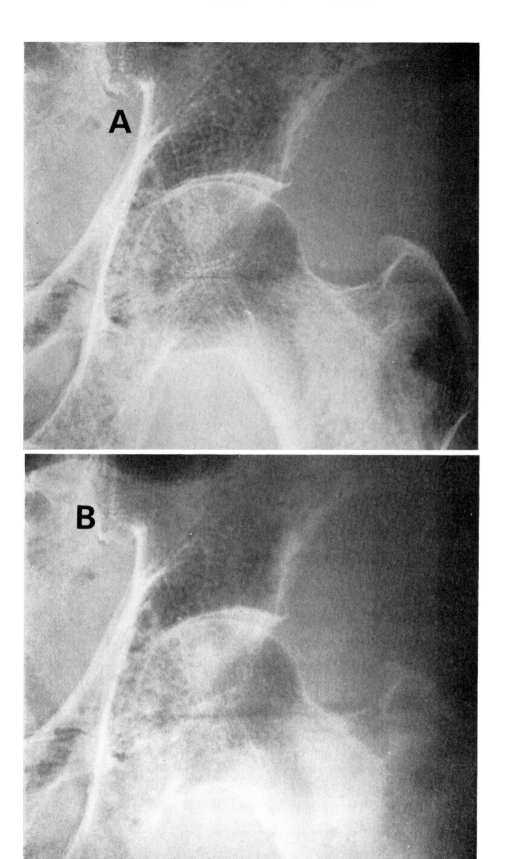

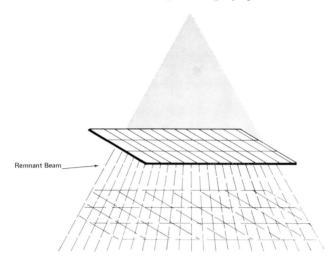

Figure 198. Additional evidence that there are indeed two separate components to the x-ray beam: (1) the projected or geometric image as seen here and (2) the variation in beam intensity and quantity which can be called the technical beam.

In practice, the radiologic technologist should develop a similar regimen with film critique that can be followed easily and quickly but at the same time provide enough information so that important observations are not overlooked. The remaining part of this chapter will deal with the problem of establishing a fixed regimen for critiquing a film and to present some actual examples of radiographs with technical problems to show how effective this method can be to help identify a technical problem and make a decision as to the correct technical adjustment.

There are three basic steps involved in this approach to film critique. The first step is the determination as to whether the radiographic problem is that of definition of detail or visibility of detail, the second is to determine the cause of the problem; the third is to choose the appropriate corrective action.

How to Identify a Definition Problem

Before going any further, it would be valuable to gain an understanding as to how these definition problems may present themselves in the radiographic image. Definition problems will usually manifest as blurring, although shape and size distortion can also be frequently seen. Magnification most often occurs when doing portables, operating room procedures, or off-table grid work, and often cannot be corrected entirely because of the nature of the situation. Sometimes blurring can be so uniform that it is difficult to notice because of the lack of any neighboring sharp lines with which comparisons can be made, so the technologist must be careful not to overlook this subtle but important problem. Figure 199A shows the problem of such a blurring situation. Most often it appears in chest films because of the patient's involuntary motion. In fact, the most frequent cause of blurring is patient motion, and the second is poor screen contact. Figure 199B is the same patient using a quicker exposure and observing the patient with more care while the exposure is being made. The difference by comparison is obvious yet if the blurred film were viewed alone and one was not trained to look for this problem it might very well not be picked up.

Causes for Blurring

The focal spot size influences sharpness or blurring of the radiographic image. The focal spot or target is, of course, where the beam originates. Many photons coming from different areas of the focal spot pass through the same body part but in slightly different directions, causing a kind of criss-crossing action. Only a little imagination is needed to understand how this would affect an examination of a complex structure such as the lung fields of the chest. Thus, one should use the smallest focal spot possible. When object film distance is increased, enlargement (magnification) occurs of all body parts including blurring itself. Figure 200 shows one film taken at a normal object film distance. Also note that the object film distance of the immediate structure under examination increases with increasing angles of the x-ray tube. In summary, problems with definition of detail are caused by how the beam is projected through the patient and eventually to the film. Screens complicate the projection problem even further under normal conditions by emitting divergent light patterns from each crystal, and if film screen contact is poor, the projection of the screen's light rays makes blurring even more obvious. Please note the outline below regarding *probable* causes for definition of detail problems.

Definition of Detail (Projection)

Problems	Causes
Blurring	Patient motion
	Screens
	Large focal spot
	O.F.D.
	Acute C.R. angle
Size Distortion	Long O.F.D.
	Short F.F.D.
Shape Distortion	Angled C.R.
	Angled film

Causes of Problems in Visibility of Detail

It is entirely possible that a radiograph with poor density or contrast characteristics could result from one of a number of items, including outdated film, processing problems, defective grids, screens, etc. To further

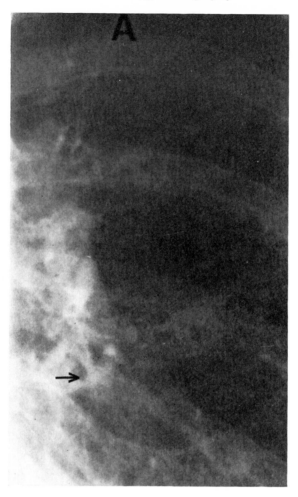

illustrate the complexity of the situation, it is important for the technologist to be able to organize these items mentally while critiquing a film for technical quality so the possibilities of making the correct adjustment will be significantly increased. For example, in the case of a radiograph that looks too light one should be able to determine whether the problem is because of insufficient quantity of radiation or because of insufficient penetration. Each of these problems requires different corrective action. The light film could also be caused by inactive developer solution, perhaps through poor replenishment rates or low temperature. The poor density might be the result of an improperly used grid resulting in grid cutoff. On the other hand, the light film might have been caused by pathology in the patient. An equal number of possibilities would be present if we were looking at a radiograph that was too dark.

When diagnosing poor contrast, a similar number of possibilities loom.

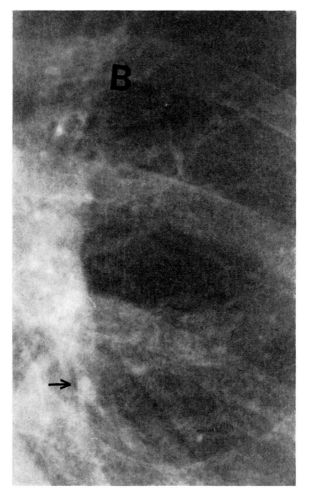

← Figure 199. Although there may appear to be only subtle differences in blurring, small fracture lines, small vessels in an arteriogram study, or small bone trabeculi would be almost impossible to see.

A flat gray-looking film could be caused by too high a Kv that produced homogenic penetration of the body part and increased the number of scatter photons. It is a possibility that the developer is too inactive (weak) to reduce the exposed silver bromide crystal properly. The grid ratio might be too low allowing excess numbers of scatter to reach the film. The developer solution might also have been too warm causing indiscriminate reduction of the unexposed crystals producing unwanted densities (chemical fog). The film might be outdated or stored for a time in too warm an area. The patient may simply have very little subject contrast and predictably a low radiographic contrast would result. As

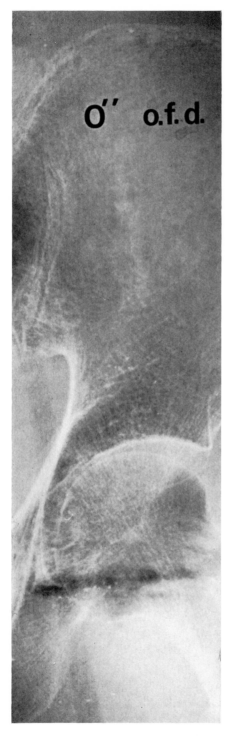

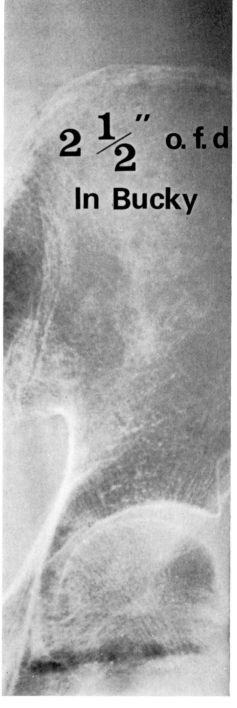

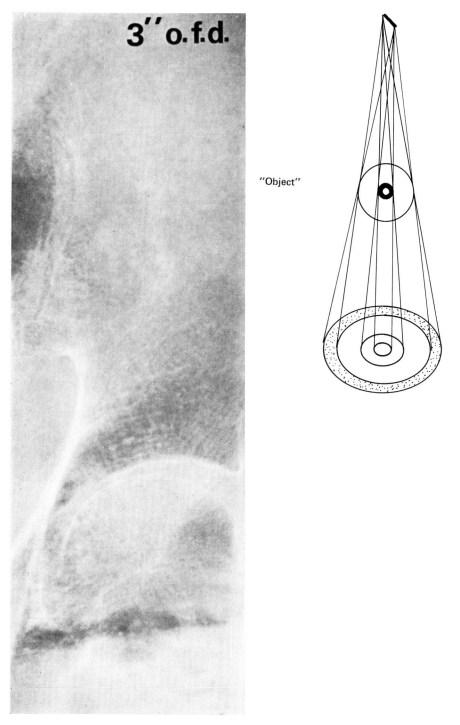

3″ o.f.d.

"Object"

← Figure 200. As object film distance increases, there is a notable decrease in sharpness of the borders of body parts to the point where they cannot be distinguished from the surrounding area.

these items come to mind, the technologist must be successful at diagnosing the problem so that the proper adjustment can be made for the repeat film. In short, the film must be analyzed technically by establishing an organized logical outline which progressively reduces the possibilities of causes and eventually will help us arrive at which factor actually caused the poor image.

The Correct Procedure

The three steps used in film critique are the following (see also Fig. 201): (1) Identify the problem; (2) Determine the cause of the problem; (3) Choose the appropriate corrective action. The first step is to determine whether or not the problem is that of definition or that of visibility of detail.

AN EFFECTIVE APPROACH TO FILM CRITIQUE

STEP ONE Determine whether you are observing a visibility problem or a projection problem

STEP TWO Review the status of the image regarding the eight items below:

Projection Problems 1. Blurring
2. Distortion of
—size
—shape

Visibility Problems 3. Artifacts
4. Body habitus
5. Contrast
6. Density
7. Penetration
8. Processing

STEP THREE (A) Determine the correction
(See Table IV)

(B) Choose the new exposure factors
(See Chapter 11)

Figure 201. The three primary steps for film critique.

The second step in film critique is to mentally review the items that are likely to cause problems with either definition or visibility of detail. For example, if the problem is a definition problem we might want to look at exposure time because of patient blurring or perhaps we would examine a cassette for poor screen contact. The eight categories in Figure 201 can be memorized quite easily if arranged in alphabetical order. After reviewing this list mentally, and keeping in mind the information discussed in previous chapters, you should be able to tell whether you are dealing with a visibility problem of a definition problem, and determine the root cause of the problem.

We must then go to step 3 to determine which course of action is most likely to correct the problem, including the choice of new exposure factors.

With the information previously given, it is possible to determine which adjustments should be made to correct the appearance of the radiographic image, i.e. whether the KvP should be adjusted, whether to use a higher or lower grid ratio, or whether the temperature of the developing solution is incorrect. Once the decision has been made, the actual exposure factors that are to be used can be obtained with the information given in Chapter Eleven. Thus, the final step to be taken in our established film critique procedure is to actually decide on which of the items in step 2 need to be corrected. This can be done successfully only if you know how far the original radiograph is from what is desired. For example, assuming the radiograph is too light and a simple adjustment in MaS is needed, before one can choose the new exposure factors he must know how light the image really is. He must be able to say to himself the radiograph is one-half the density it should be or perhaps it is three-quarters the density it should be.

If the film is one-half the desired density the exposure factors must be increased by two times or doubled, but if the image is approximately 75 percent of the density which is desired, the exposure must be increased by 25 percent. Another situation may be that the image is too low in contrast, which of course could be the result of a number of problems. It might be because the exposure produced too many scatter photons causing radiographic fog. It might also be a problem of poor subject contrast as a result of an old patient with very poor absorption tissue characteristics. In this case we will assume that the KvP is to be reduced to help increase subject contrast. The next step is to choose the correct KvP that will provide the desired effect. It has been the author's experience that a reduction in KvP to increase subject contrast requires an adjustment of at least 15 to 20 KvP. This, of course, would reduce radiographic density and so the MaS must be increased accordingly. However, before such an adjustment is made, once again the technologist must ask himself specifically how much of a kilovoltage decrease is necessary to cause the desired effect. A fairly accurate estimate must be made as to how this change will affect density; by reviewing Chapter Eleven, the correct adjustment can be made with relative ease.

We will now critique two examinations using our three-step film critique procedure. Refer to Figure 202: Here we have a technical prob-

TABLE IV

POSSIBLE REMEDIES FOR POOR RADIOGRAPHIC QUALITY

General Radiographic Problem	Specific Radiographic Problem	Possible Solutions
Artifacts	foreign body in screens	These generally show as white marks on the film. Cassette screens should be replaced if the surface is pitted.
	static	Try to increase humidity. Use a fine mist to spray walls of darkroom. Use antistatic solution on screens during the static season (winter).
	fingerprints	Try to reduce moisture on hands. Occasional washing or cleansing with alcohol soaked cotton balls will help. Avoid contact with film except on edges.
	scratches	These can result from dirty rollers and/or misadjusted guide shoes; occasionally, too much pressure when feeding film will cause tiny plus density scratches. Usually, processor scratches will be in the direction of film travel.
Blurring	patient motion	Use compression, restraints, shorter exposures. Reduce to at least 1/10 or 1/15 of a second for adults, 1/120 of a second for children. Use super-high speed screens. Reduce F.F.D. only if absolutely necessary. Use lower ratio grid.
	poor film contact	Do a screen test. New felt straps or hinges might be needed. Replace cassette if frame is warped.
	too much O.F.D.	Increase F.F.D. if possible.
Poor Contrast	excessive S/S radiation	There are many ways to reduce S/S radiation reaching the film. All, however, become more or less desirable depending on the particular situation. One must not lower the KvP at the risk of inadequate penetration. The formula for finding optimal KvP can be used as a guide.
		Coning is very important as shown in Chapter Nine. With flabby patients, compression can be very helpful. Of course, increasing grid ratio will absorb extra S/S. One should keep in mind that flabby, fat patients often do not require nearly the MaS or KvP that is indicated on the chart through mere cm measurement. This type of patient requires a reduction in KvP to yield positive results. Muscular people, of course, often require more KvP than indicated by measurement. Even with muscular people, the base KvP formula will usually be sufficient.
	chemical fog	Chemical fog is the result of overactive developer solution. There are three ways to correct the situation. If processor is overreplenishing, reset the switches. Often the incoming water temperature will rise and cause the developing tank to overheat through conduction; reduce water temperature to approximately 60 degrees for quick cooling and readjust to 85 for routine operation. Also check

TABLE IV *(Continued)*

POSSIBLE REMEDIES FOR POOR RADIOGRAPHIC QUALITY

General Radiographic Problem	Specific Radiographic Problem	Possible Solutions
		for exhausted solution or improperly mixed developer solution. Inactive developer will produce poor contrast. Basically the same factors that affect developer activity must be reviewed: developer replenisher, temperature, and one additional factor, oxidation. If too low, increase replenisher rate to at least 100 cc of fixer per 14 × 17 and 55 cc developer per 14 × 17. In low volume areas these rates should be as much as 50 percent higher. Consult the chapter on automatic processing. The developer temperature should be increased to 92–95°. If the developer is oxidized, new solution must be mixed.
	body habitus	Subject contrast relates directly to radiographic contrast. If the patient is elderly and dehydrated with poor muscle tone, reduce the KvP by *at least* 10 to 15 and adjust MaS for density. Certain pathologies require KvP adjustments. These are so varied that space does not allow a detailed description. One should know which diseases cause tissue to break down, requiring lower KvP. For muscular patients, you are forced to use at least base KvP. Very little can be done in these cases except to use a heavier grid and careful coning.
	film fog	Occasionally, film will be stored incorrectly, resulting in high levels of base fog and mottle. One must check the film's base fog if poor storage conditions are a possibility.
Density	exposure factors	Through experience one must develop an intuition about the exposure factor used for the body type and related situation (grid/screens/film etc.). Over penetration might be part of the problem. Excessive developer temperature, over replenishment, or simply too much MaS could be the problem. The wrong film or screen may have been used. As we will see later, the general appearance of the film as well as background information must be used to review all possible causes. Most often, it is a matter of over penetration and/or too much MaS.
Distortion	angulation of body or CR increased O.F.D.	This probably occurs most when doing portable work. One must be sure to position the body part correctly with the appropriate angle of CR. When the object film distance is increased, the F.F.D. should be increased proportionately. Maintain an acceptable ratio of O.F.D. to F.F.D. whenever possible, i.e. 2.0 inch O.F.D. to 40 inch F.F.D. or 3 inch O.F.D. to 60 inch F.F.D.
Patient	elderly patients	Often, body habitus has a very strong influence on the appearance of the radiographic image. Elderly patients have a very low hydration level which decreases subject contrast

TABLE IV (*Continued*)

POSSIBLE REMEDIES FOR POOR RADIOGRAPHIC QUALITY

General Radiographic Problem	Specific Radiographic Problem	Possible Solutions
		greatly. Use a beam that will produce more photoelectric interactions, which would improve or amplify the existing poor subject contrast (decrease KvP 15 to 20 KvP).
	demineralized bone	Occasionally, the bones of elderly people become demineralized and thus offer little stopping power to the beam. The bones on radiographs look almost as dark as the surrounding soft tissue, which produces even less subject contrast (lower KvP by 15 to 20 KvP).
	muscular patients	Another problem relative to body habitus is when the patient has very firmly developed muscle tissue. The water content in this case is high which makes penetration difficult and, in addition, produces an excess of S/S radiation. Both situations combined cause a light and very low contrast radiographic image. The solution is difficult, because the increase in KvP needed to penetrate the highly absorbent muscle tissue helps produce an increased scatter ratio. A very careful balance of KvP and MaS is needed. Extra grid ratio is helpful. Sometimes using a grid cassette in a bucky will help in extreme cases. The use of rare earth screens sometimes can compromise for a decrease in KvP. Proper coning is important as well.
	obese patients	Patients with a high fat content often produce a very flat, gray looking film. One should keep in mind that fatty tissue is easily penetrated and, although the physical size of the patient is great, one can often reduce the KvP by ten and not loose too much density. This would also reduce the ratio of S/S production producing a higher contrast image. Finally, compression can be used with some degree of success. Very often, radiographs of fat patients are simply over exposed and a reduction of technique in general, preferably in KvP, will produce a better image. Coning is important also.
Penetration	too thick or dense body tissue (too much absorption)	It is very difficult for untrained technologists to determine whether under or over penetration is the problem. Too little penetration produces an image that has poor contrast with very light density. The bony parts when viewed are almost undistinguishable, as they have very similar density to the surrounding soft tissue. An increase of at least 10 to 15 KvP is usually necessary. Increasing by 20 KvP is sometimes indicated in extreme cases. Coning is important to help reduce S/S as much as possible.
	too little absorption	The solution and resulting image is more successful than with the above condition. Here one may reduce the KvP by 15 and in extreme cases by 20. One must be careful, of course, not to use a KvP that will produce inadequate penetration.

TABLE IV (*Continued*)

POSSIBLE REMEDIES FOR POOR RADIOGRAPHIC QUALITY

General Radiographic Problem	Specific Radiographic Problem	Possible Solutions
Processing	chemical fog (overactive developer)	Chemical fog occurs when the reducing agents begin to work on the unexposed silver bromide crystals. This produces an over-all density in areas of the film that are supposed to be white. Check for high developer temperature. The easiest way to identify chemical fog is to look at the area of the film containing the patient's name and x-ray number. If it appears gray, then it is probably caused by overactive or contaminated developer. Also, the replenishing rates should be checked for possible replenishment.
	underactive developer	This situation produces an image with very little contrast and low density. The film usually has a "washed out" look. Too low a developer activity is usually the cause. The solution is simple once the cause is determined. The developer temperature for automatic, 90 sec processing should be about 95°. Replenishment should be about 55 cc per 14 × 17 film (developer), and if the solution is exhausted and oxidized it must be replaced with fresh solution. Check for diluted developer.

lem with poor contrast and increased density. The patient was to have an IVP examination, and the scout film is very dark and extremely low in contrast. The patient measured 26 cm and was quite flabby. As you can see from looking at the scout film (A), a major adjustment in technique is necessary. The lack of contrast makes it impossible to see any detail whatever.

Our first step in film critique is to determine whether we are dealing with a definition of detail problem or a visibility of detail problem. The structures appear to be sharp; upon close inspection of the radiograph, the bone markings of the pelvis appear to be well defined, and since there is no evidence of distortion we can direct our attention to the factors involving visibility of detail. We can now review the six items under visibility of detail which would help us isolate the problem still further. Artifacts can be eliminated immediately. Body habitus is certainly a problem because of the patient's size and fat content. Contrast is certainly too low, and there is too much density on the film. At first the film appears to be overpenetrated, but the KvP used was 90 and this would not cause overpenetration of a part of a patient of this size. Processing does not appear to be the problem because the patient's identification name plate has good image characteristics. (Fig. 201 shows a checklist that can be used in the classroom.) Also, the other films processed at the same time looked normal. Thus, with step 2, we have eliminated more possibilities and have come

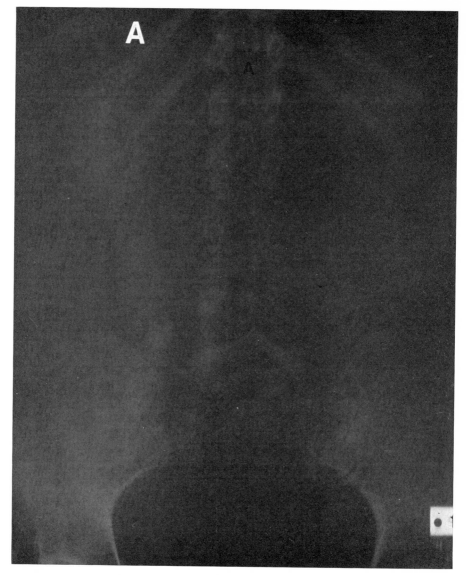

Figure 202A.

Figure 202. By using an established, logical, simple approach, film critique can be accomplished easily. Proper use of the various conversion factors will help make step 3 easier.

closer to the root of the problem. It appears in summary that the patient is the basic problem because of his body habitus, but because of the factors used, contrast and density were unacceptable. Although this may seem obvious, the established procedure or regimen helped us to review

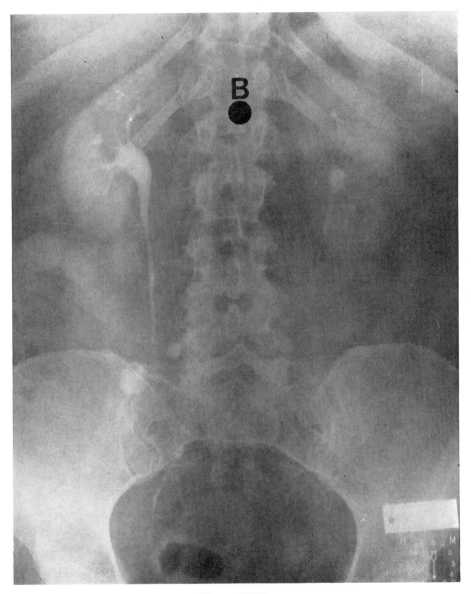

Figure 202B.

and eliminate many other problems very quickly that *could have* contributed to this situation.

The third step in our program requires us to review all of the items in step 3 that involve body habitus. We may also wish to review the sections on radiographic contrast and density for additional information that may help us decide on the most appropriate corrective action. The original technique was 400 Ma, one second at 90 KvP. We estimate through

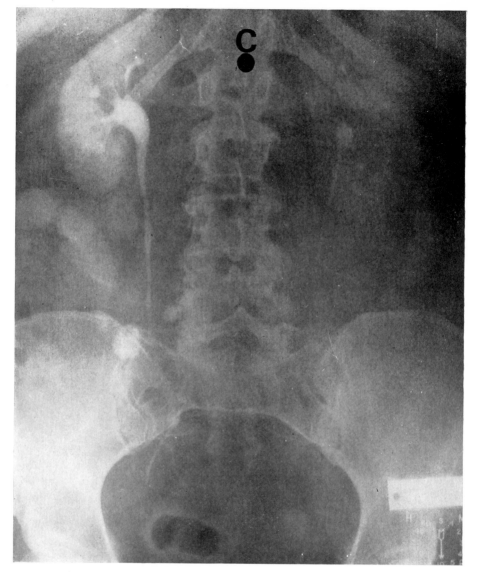

Figure 202C.

experience that the density is approximately four times darker than it should be and reduce the exposure to one quarter and obtain film B. We note, however, that the contrast is still low because of poor subject contrast and probably excess scatter as well. We know subject contrast can be improved by decreasing KvP, also less scatter will be produced. We know further that a reduction in KvP of 15 percent will reduce radiographic density by one-half. With this in mind, the third film was exposed using 76 KvP at one-half second and the results are noted in film C. Thus,

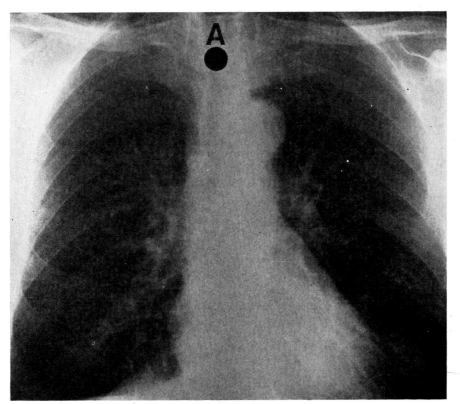

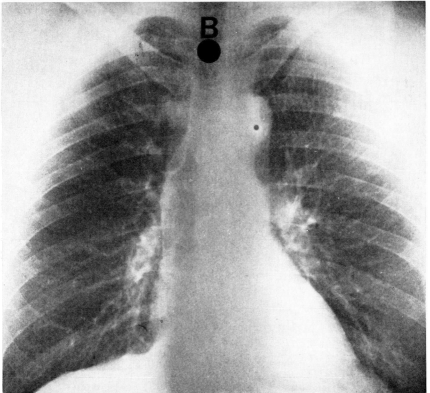

Figure 203.

by using the three step system we have effectively, without skipping any important factors, reviewed many possibilities and systematically came to the conclusion that subject contrast and overexposure were the primary problems. By using the information presented in Chapter Eleven, we were able to make the necessary conversions and affect the optimal image for that particular patient's examination.

A chest examination is shown in Figure 203. By inspection of film A we note that there is a great deal of density. There is no evidence of distortion or blurring so we can once again direct our attention away from those factors that affect definition of detail and distortion. As we go down the list of six categories listed in step 2, all can be eliminated quickly except for excessive density and possibly overpenetration. At first one might suspect overpenetration (too much Kv for a given body part) but it is very common to use 110 KvP for grid chest studies. This leaves us with a simple case of overexposure as a result of too much MaS. We must now look again at film A and determine how much darker it is over what we consider optimal and in this case we decide the image is approximately two times darker than it should be. The exposure time was thus reduced by one-half and the results of the second exposure can be noted in film B. The initial exposure factors were 300 Ma, 110 KvP at $\frac{1}{15}$ second. The final exposure used was 300 Ma, 110 KvP at $\frac{1}{30}$th of a second.

BIBLIOGRAPHY

Cahoon: *Formulating X-Ray Techniques.* North Carolina, Duke Printing, 1970.

Cleare, Splettstosser Seemann: Experimental Study of the Mottle Produced by X-Ray Intensifying Screens. *AJR*, No. 1:168-174, July 1962.

Cullinan: Illustrated Guide to X-Ray Technics. Philadelphia, Lippincott, 1972.

Curry III; Nunnally: *Introduction to the Physics of Diagnostic Radiography.* Philadelphia, Lea & Febiger, 1972.

Fuchs: *Principles of Radiographic Exposure Processing.* Springfield, Thomas, 1972.

Funke: Illumination. *Picker Corp.,* Vol. 18(3):2-22.

Hodes, Jacque DeMoor, Ernst: Body Section Radiography: Fundamentals. *Radiol. Clinic North Am.,* April, pp. 229-242.

Liebel, Flarsheim: *Characteristics and Applications of X-Ray Grids.* Cincinnati, 1968.

Lundh: Film Fogging by Radiation From Building Materials. *Photographic Science & Engineering,* Liebel, Flarsheim, July 9, 1974, Reprint No. 7468.

Meredith, Massey: *Fundamental Physics of Radiography.* Baltimore, Williams & Wilkins, 1968.

Miller: *Clinical Pathology.* Baltimore, Williams & Wilkins, 1966.

Rossmann: Image Quality in Medical Radiography. *The Journal Of Photographic Science,* Vol. 12:279-283, 1964.

Seemann: *Physical & Photographic Principles of Medical Radiography.* New York, John Wiley & Sons, Inc., 1968.

Selman: *Fundamentals of X-Ray and Radium Physics.* Springfield, Thomas, 1974.

Ter-Pogossian: *Physical Aspects of Diagnostic Radiography.* New York, Harper & Row, 1969.

Trout, Dahl: *Course Manual For X-Ray Applications.* Washington, D.C., Govt. Print. Office, 1973.

Tuddenham: Physiology of Roentgen Diagnosis. *AJAR,* Vol. LXXVIII, No. 1:116-123, July 1957.

Webb: Number of Quanta Required to Form the Photographic Latent Image. *Journal Optical Society of America.* Vol. 31, No. 9:559-569, Sept. 1941.

INDEX

A

Absorption
  effect of body habitus, 200, 201, 202
  effect of KvP, 178, 179
  effect of pathology, 200, 216
  variation of absorption, 8, 225, 229
Air gap, 161, 163
Angulation of tube, 165, 332
Anode, 175
  focal spot size, 115
  heat loading, 112, 113
  high speed, 144
  rotating, 114, 144
  stationary, 114
Anode heel effect, 170, 171, 172
Artifacts
  processor, 56-60
  screen, 97-98, 100
Automatic processing, 47-49
  advantages of, 48
  agents, chemical, 44
  artifacts, 56, 100
  centralized, 48
  chemical activity, 12
  chemical fog, 26, 46, 52, 67, 335
  dispersal, 48
  drying system, 65
  important considerations, 51
  maintenance, 74
  margin for error, 54
  reaction particles, 52, 55, 56, 57
  recirculating system, 66
  replenishment rates, 63, 64, 65
  replenishment system, 57
  trouble shooting, 69, 70-74
Autotransformer, 177, 178
Average gradient, 25

B

Background radiation, 32
Base plus fog, 26, 32, 37, 75
Beam, x-ray
  absorption distribution, 183, 184, 201
  characteristics of, 183
  efficiency, 189
  heterogenic, 179, 182, 183, 184
  homogenic, 182, 183, 184, 199
  monochromatic, 179, 182, 183, 184
  polychromatic, 179, 182, 183, 184
  projected, 133, 134
  restriction devices, 235, 240
  technical, 133
Body (see also Habitus)
  abdomen, 201, 217
  absorption characteristics, 225, 265
  bone content, 202, 212
  chest, 182, 217
  evaluation of, 201, 202, 214
  extremities, 219
  fat, 202, 205, 206
  fluid, 217
  motion, 333
  muscle, 202, 207
  regions of, 217
  skull, 220
Bucky assembly, 260, 261
  installation, 260, 261

C

Calcium tungstate, 80, 81
Carboard exposures, 35, 36
Cassettes
  grid, 269
Cathode, 175
Characteristic curve, 18
  contrast, 21
  latitude, 22
Characteristic radiation, 223
Chemical activity, 12
Chemical agents, 44
Chemical fog, 26, 46, 52, 67, 335
Circuit, 111, 112, 177, 178
  filament, 110
  primary, 111, 112
  secondary, 177, 178
Coating, film, 35, 36
Collimators, 235, 237, 240
  effect on density and contrast, 235, 240
  effect on patient dose, 242
  effect on scatter, 235, 240
Compression, mark, 60
Compton effect, 221, 227
  controlling factor, 192, 227
  effect on contrast, 192

effect on remnant beam, 8, 13, 16, 184, 221
effect on scatter production, 192

D

Darkroom, 47, 48
Decentering, 134, 160, 161
  grid, 261
  projected image, 134, 135
Definition of detail, 332
Density, 6, 7, 12, 13, 15, 34, 38, 42, 57, 68
  diagnostic range, 18, 25, 324
Detail, 5, 18, 24
  sharpness of, 15, 16, 329
  visibility of, 5, 15, 16, 37, 326
Developing agents, 43, 44
Developing time, 41, 42
Diagnostic quality, 6, 29
Diaphragm, 235, 240
Differential absorption, 8
Direct exposure, 29, 76, 109
Distance, FFD, 133, 134, 144
  effect on contrast, 137
  effect on density, 133, 134, 138, 140
  effect on sharpness, 144, 158, 159, 170
  finding correct FFD, 137
  short FFD, 157
Distortion
  parallex, 31
  shape, 165, 332
  size, 166, 332
Dry to dry, 49
Drying system, 65

E

Electrical pressure, 174, 175
Electron cloud, 111, 112
Emphysema, 216
Emulsion (*see also* Film)
  thickness, 34, 35, 36, 52
Energy conversion
  into x-rays, 111, 112, 174, 176

F

Fat, 204
  absorption, 204, 206
  effect on radiographic contrast, 204
  effect on subject contrast, 206
Field size, 134, 235, 236
  patient dose, 242
Filament
  circuit, 110, 111, 177
  incandescence, 112
  space charge, 111, 112, 113
  tube current, 111, 113, 174, 175

Film, 27
  absorption of x-rays, 76
  automatic processing, 52
  base, 26, 30, 32, 75
  coating, 35, 36
  construction, 28
  contrast, 8, 9, 10, 15, 21, 24, 35
  crystal, 13, 32, 33, 34, 38
  double coating, 36
  emulsion, 29, 34, 35
  feeding, 64
  gelatin, 35, 36
  glass plate, 27
  grain, 33, 34
  latitude, 35
  nonscreen, 29, 76, 109
  parallex, 31
  screen, 29, 32, 33, 36, 77, 109
  sensitivity to x-ray, 32, 33, 34
  sensitivity to pressure, 59, 60
  storage, 37
Film critique, 323
  approach to, 330-338
  diagnosing technical problems, 322, 340-343
Filtration, 229
  added, 230
  effect on beam, 230
  effect on image, 230
  effect on patient dose, 229, 231
  inherent, 229
  total, 230
Fixed KvP
  technique chart, 197, 198
Fixer, 43, 44 (*see also* Processing)
Fluid body, 202, 207, 217
Fluorescence, 81
  color of emission, 76, 77
  definition, 76, 77, 81
  lag, 81
  processes of, 80, 81
Focal film distance, 134, 267
  effect on beam composition, 134, 136
  effect on density, 134, 136, 138
  effect on penumbra, 142, 143
  effect on sharpness, 142, 143
  inverse square law, 135, 136, 141
Focal spot
  actual focal spot, 141, 142
  effect on sharpness, 114, 115, 142, 143, 144-147
  effective focal spot, 114, 141, 142
  heat loading, 114, 116, 142
  line focus principle, 141, 142

magnification, 157, 158
point source, 142
rotating, 114, 141, 142, 144
size, 114, 115, 142, 144, 146
stationary, 114
Fog
base plus fog, 32, 45
chemical, 45, 46, 52
effect on contrast, 46, 204, 243
effect on detail, 45, 46
effect on visibility, 45, 46
Fractional focal spot, 144

G

Generator, 111, 112, 178
Glass plates, 27
Gradient average, 22-25
Grain, film, 33, 34
Green light emission, 76, 77
Grid, 243
absorption of beam, 243, 245, 266
bucky assembly, 260
cassette, 269
clean up, 244, 245, 266
construction, 244
conversion in exposure, 242, 320
cross, 248, 253, 256
cut off, 247, 248, 249, 251, 253
decentering, 261
effect on contrast, 261
effect on density, 261
effect on scatter, 191, 244, 263, 266
efficiency, 245, 256
fine line, 260, 268
focused, 249, 253, 256, 257
linear, 249, 256
materials used, 260
microline, 260, 268
parallel, 249
patient dose, 242
positioning latitude, 244, 249, 266
ratio, 244, 245, 249, 266
selection of, 245, 263, 264, 266, 269
selectivity, 256

H

H & D curve, 18
average gradient, 22, 23, 25
contrast film, 18, 21, 24
diagnostic range, 25
latitude, 22
location, 21
shape, 21, 22
shoulder, 18

speed film, 21
toe, 18
Habitus, 200, 201
age of patient, 207, 213
bone content, 202, 212
effect on absorption, 197, 206, 225
effect on exposure values, 206
effect on radiographic contrast, 206
effect on radiographic density, 206
evaluation of, 202, 214
fat, 202, 204
fluid, 202, 207, 217
muscle, 202, 207
pathology, 200, 201-205, 216
Heat
anode, 113, 115, 126, 144, 198
contributing factors, *see* Focal spot size
dispersal in tube, 127, 141
limitations of, 141, 144
Heat exchanger, 67
Heel effect, 170, 171, 172
High KvP technique, 184
Hypo solution, 44

I

Image, radiographic characteristics, 16, 38
contrast, 3, 4, 6, 8, 15, 16
density, 3, 4, 12, 13, 15, 16, 114
diagnostic, 3, 38
latent, 37, 38, 41
projected, 38
radiographic, 29, 38
sharpness, 142
technical, 38
Incandescence, 112
Inherent filtration, 84, 86
Intensification factor, 84, 85, 86
Intensity, beam, 12, 13, 127, 134, 136, 137
effect on contrast, 15, 16
effect on density, 15, 16, 134
Intensifying screens, 76
active layer, 80
advantages of, 77
artifacts, 97, 98
backing, 77
classification of, 84, 85, 86
color light emission, 76, 77, 98
construction, 77
contact, 78, 98, 99, 102
crystal size, type, 80, 83, 84
edge seal, 80
effect on density, 86
effect on exposure, 84, 85, 86
effect on patient dose, 77, 84, 85

effect on sharpness, 76, 84, 87, 89, 91, 96
exposure efficiency, 76, 77, 82, 86
film, 36, 85
fluorescence, 76, 77, 80, 81
lag, 100
light emission, 80, 90
maintenance, 105
milliamperage, 110 (*see also* Luminescence)
modulation transfer function, 87, 90, 97
mottle, 103, 105
noise, 103
protective layer, 80
primary, 16, 178
rare earth, 105-108
reflective layer, 78, 79, 94
remnant, 8, 10
speed, 82, 84, 86, 93
unsharpness, 79, 84, 86, 87, 89, 96
variation of intensity, 182, 183, 188, 197
Inverse square law, 134, 136, 141, 144
causes, 136
effect on density, 134, 136
effect on exposure factors, 136
Ions, 38, 39, 40

K

Kilovoltage
base KvP, 193
beam efficiency, 179, 188, 189
beam quality, 178, 188
beam quantity, 178
circuit, 177
control of, 178
conversion, 319 (Table)
conversion of kinetic energy, 175, 176
effect on beam, 179, 183, 184
effect on contrast (radiographic), 191, 192,
193, 216, 221
effect on density (radiographic), 193
effect on fog, 191, 192
effect on patient dose, 188, 189
effect on penetration, 178
exposure latitude, 183, 184, 185, 186, 187
fifteen percent rule, 186, 314
fixed KvP, 196, 197, 198
grid selection, 263, 269
high KvP, 184
interactions, 188, 189, 192, 193, 196, 221,
226, 227
mottle, 104
optimal, 197, 198
selection of, 192, 193, 196, 198
subject contrast, 182, 183, 196, 197
tube loading, 179, 188, 189, 198

variable KvP, 197, 198
wavelength, 179

L

Lag, screen, 100
Latent image, 37, 38, 41, 43
Latitude
exposure, 183, 184
film, 22-35
positioning, 244, 249, 266
Lattice, crystal, 38, 40
Line focus principle, 141
Luminescence, 76
calibration, 117
conversion, 318-320 (Table)
definition, 110
effect on contrast, 123, 124
effect on density, 114, 122
exposure rate, 119
heat generated, 113, 198
milliamperage, 110
milliampere-seconds, 117, 118, 121, 171,
178, 207
patient dose, 119
quantity of primary rays, 178
selection of, 110, 112, 113
sharpness of detail, 115

M

Magnification, 157, 158
advantages, 164
controlling factors, 158
effect on penumbra, 144, 164
fractional focal spot, 157
size distortion, 166
Magnification technique, 157, 163
advantages, 157
causes, 160
prerequisites for, 157, 158
Mammography, 12
Meters
KvP, 178
Ma, 113, 119, 178
MaS, 119
Modulation transfer function, 97, 108
Motion
control of patients, 115
Mottle
quantum, 103-104
screen, 103-104
Muscle (*see* Body *and* Habitus)

N

Noise screen (*see* Mottle)

O

Object film distance, 140, 143, 152, 157, 162, 166
  advantages of, 157, 164
  controlling factors, 158
  disadvantages of, 144, 164
  effect on contrast, 161, 163
  effect on density, 161, 163
  effect on scatter, 163
  effect on sharpness, 142, 143
  effect on size distortion, 152, 157, 158
  penumbra, 142, 143
Overdevelopment, 57
Overreplenishment, 57

P

Paget's disease, 203
Parallex distortion, 31
Pathology, 200, 216
Patient x-ray absorption, 200 (*see also* Body *and* Habitus)
Penetration of x-rays, 176, 179, (*see also* Kilovoltage)
  controlling factors, 177, 179
Penumbra, 144, 152, 157
  causes, 142, 143
  control of, 144, 157
  definition, 142
Phosphorescence, 81, 82, 83, 100
Phosphors, 76
Photoelectric cell, 128
Photoelectric interaction, 192, 193, 221, 226
Photon, light, screens, 81
Photon, primary, 16, 178
Photon, remnant, 8, 13, 15, 16, 184, 221
Photon, scatter, 192
Phototiming, 128, 200
  advantages, 128, 129, 132
  back-up timer, 130
  disadvantages, 122, 129, 130
  positioning body part, 129, 130, 131
  reaction time, 129
Pi lines, 56
Planography (*see* tomography)
Plesiotomography, 285
Point source, 142
Polychromatic beam, 179, 183, 184
Polyenergetic beam, 179, 183, 184
Potential, current, 175, 176
Primary x-rays, 16, 178
Processing, 47 (*see also* Automatic processing)
  artifacts, 56-60
  automatic, 49
  base fog, 75

chemical fog, 52, 67
developing agents, 44
drying system, 65
exhausted solutions, 57, 61, 62
film type, 51, 52
fixing agents, 44
heat exchanger, 67
maintenance, 74
manual, 47, 48
overdevelopment, 57, 63, 64, 65
overreplenishment, 57, 63, 64, 65
recirculating system, 66
replenishment system, 57, 65
temperature developer, 52, 67
temperature time processing, 67, 68
temperature, water, 67
transport system, 36, 53-57
underdevelopment, 57, 62
underreplenishment, 62
Projected image, 133

Q

Quality of beam, (*see also* Kilovoltage)
  image, 6, 29
Quantum, 104, 179
Quantum mottle, 103, 106, 107
Quantum theory, 104, 179

R

Radiation
  absorption, 183, 184, 189
  characteristic, 179, 183, 184
  efficiency, 179, 188, 189
  energy of, 176, 179
  frequency, 179
  primary, 16, 178
  production of, 112, 173, 176
  quantum, 103, 104
  remnant, 8, 13, 15, 16, 184, 221
Radiograph, 3
  contrast, 6, 7, 8, 10, 12, 57, 61, 62, 89, 137, 164
  density, 34, 57, 62, 68, 134, 136, 228
  detail, 18, 24, 114
  image, 15
  sharpness, 78, 79, 89
Ratio, grid, 244 (*see also* Grid)
Reaction particles, 52, 67
Reaction time, 129
Reciprocating bucky, 260
Reciprocity law, 115, 116
Recoil electron, 227
Reducing agents, 41, 43

Remnant beam, 15, 226
Replenishment
    overreplenishment, 57, 63, 64, 65
    replenishment rates, 65
    underreplenishment, 62
Roentgen, 3
Roentgenogram, 3
Rotating anode, 144

S

Safelights, 50
Scatter, 164, 191, 217, 235, 243, 245
    compton effect on, 227
    control of, 163, 191, 244, 245
    effect on contrast, 193, 228, 235, 261, 263
    effect on density, 191, 193, 236, 261
Secondary radiation
Sensitivity speck, 37-39, 40, 41
Sensitometor, 75
Sensitometry, 18
    diagnostic range, 18
Shape distortion, 165
Sharpness, 6
    detail, 15, 16, 329
Silver bromide crystal
    absorption to x-ray, 76, 77
    accumulation, 7, 13, 33, 38
    effect on contrast, 24, 33, 34
    effect on density, 6, 8, 10, 13, 14
    effect on film speed, 33, 34
    shape of, 32, 34
    size of, 32, 33, 34
Soft radiation, 230
Space charge, 111, 112, 113
Static, 99
Stationary anode, 114
Subject contrast, 6, 8, 10, 12, 193, 206, 209,
    217, 218, 225, 226

T

Target area, 115, 152
    loading, 114, 115
    shape, 114
    size, 114, 115
Technical beam, 133
Technique charts, 199

exposure time, 129
    fixed KvP, 197, 198
    optimal KvP, 197, 198
    variable KvP, 197, 198
Temperature
    anode, 113, 115, 126, 144, 198
    developer, 67, 68, 69
Thermionic emission, 112
Time, 115, 116, 119, 125, 127
Tomography, 270
    book cassette, 283, 287
    exposure arc, 275, 276, 293, 299, 302
    exposure, conversion, 293, 299
    exposure time, 276, 280
    exposure to patient, 285
    fulcrum, 271, 272
    ghost shadows, 282, 284
    linkage, 280, 293
    localization, 289
    multiplanography, 283, 284, 285
    objective plane, 272
        thickness of, 275, 276, 287, 299, 302
    redundant shadows, 282, 284
    zonography, 287
Tone, radiographic, 7, 8, 38
Tube current, 126, 176
Tube rating charts, 116, 126

U

Umbra, 142
Underreplenishment, 59, 62
Unsharpness, 333
    focal spot, 114, 115, 152, 162
    OFD, 140, 152, 157
    parallex, 31
    patient motion, 115
    screen, 79

V

Visibility of detail, 5, 15, 16, 39, 326
    contrast, 326, 328, 329
    density, 326
    fog, 326

W

Wavelength of x-rays, 179